NORMAL AND HANDICAPPED CHILDREN

A Growth and Development Primer
For Parents and Professionals

Wilbur S. Thain, M.D.
Glendon Casto, Ph.D.
Adrienne Peterson, R.P.T.

Exceptional Child Center
Utah State University

Illustrations by Holly Hatch

PSG Publishing Company, Inc.
Littleton, Massachusetts

Library of Congress Cataloging in Publication Data

Thain, Wilbur S
  Normal and handicapped children.

  Bibliography: p.
  Includes index.
  1. Child development.   2. Developmentally
disabled children.   3. Handicapped children.
I. Casto, Glendon, joint author.   II. Peterson,
Adrienne, joint author.   III. Title.
RJ131.T5   612.6'5   79-9402
ISBN 0-88416-227-3

Medicine is an ever-changing science. As new research and clinical experience broaden our knowledge, changes in treatment and drug therapy are required. The editors and the publisher of this work have made every effort to ensure that the treatment and drug dosage schedules herein are accurate and in accord with the standards accepted at the time of publication. Readers are advised, however, to check the product information sheet included in the package of each drug they plan to administer to be certain that changes have not been made in the recommended dose or in the indications and contraindications for administration. This recommendation is of particular importance in regard to new or infrequently used drugs.

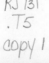

CONTENTS

"Doctor, is my baby growing the way he should?"

"Why is Jeremy so much smaller than his older brother was at two years of age?"

"Doctor, I'm worried! My father-in-law says my baby is a mongoloid. Is he?"

"The neighbor says my baby may be retarded because he doesn't use his left arm. He doesn't act retarded, Doctor, but why doesn't he use his arm?"

These are the types of actual questions which have instigated the development and production of this book. It is the authors' desire to attempt to discuss and describe the average growth and development of children in a way that is understandable to nonprofessional people. It is also our hope to discuss briefly some of the problems of abnormal growth and development and to suggest sources where the reader might obtain help when a question arises concerning the normal development of a baby.

It is imperative that the reader realize that there are vast differences in normal development and growth. Two babies, even twins, may show differences in their growth, their weight, the ages at which they sit, crawl, walk, and talk. There are, however, guidelines which indicate that progression has fallen below normal and that problems might be arising. In these situations, it is necessary to secure professional help in evaluating the child's progress or lack of progress.

In an effort to acquaint you with what is happening in present therapy, information will be given concerning some of the broad intervention programs available in the United States today. You, as parents, should realize that these programs should be developed and outlined individually for each child then tailored to that child's specific handicap. The child must be evaluated at regular periods of time, his progress followed, and, where necessary, the program enlarged, changed, or updated.

Approaches to the prevention of defects are discussed and, where possible, recommendations as to where help can be obtained are outlined. The role of genetic counseling and prenatal diagnosis are briefly outlined and discussed.

The book will also attempt to suggest professionals, agencies, parent groups, and institutions where help might be obtained if you have a child you feel is developmentally delayed.

If you are unable to secure help, the authors and other staff members at the Exceptional Child Center at Utah State University will be happy to suggest referrals where help can be obtained.

A bibliography and glossary are included to help readers familiarize themselves with currently available materials to enable either the lay or professional person to secure more information regarding specific areas of concern.

This book does not purport to answer all the questions about the developmentally disabled. This would involve much too long and ponderous a tome—one good only to fill the bookshelf and perhaps to press butterflies or wildflowers—but of limited use to parents of growing, developing children.

This is a book written about all types of children—normal, abnormal, retarded, severely handicapped, or totally normal. Where applicable, racial differences are described, and specific genetic problems applicable to racial groups are discussed.

Specific case examples have all actually occurred within our practices and are cited to illustrate specific problems in the diagnosis and treatment of the developmentally disabled.

The authors gratefully acknowledge the assistance of Robert Wadsworth, Richard Carpenter, Vonda Douglas, and Phyllis Herr who assisted with the manuscript.

PART I

Normal Growth and Development

1   The Concept of Normality

WHAT IS A "NORMAL" CHILD?

Most parents ask themselves, at sometime or other, "Is my child normal?" They probably do not ask this question out loud. After all, there is no good reason to suspect that one's child is anything other than "Mr. Goodkid," and besides, nobody wants to sound like an over-concerned parent. But even though concerns are not voiced out loud, parents still feel them. We hope that this chapter will help answer this question.

Before one can know how normal a child is, it is necessary to under-stand the concept of normality. Pediatricians, child psychologists, or other experts on child development refer to "developmental norms" which, simply stated, tell us the age at which an "average" child acquires a certain skill or reaches a certain stage. For example, the developmental norm for taking five steps without assistance is 15 months. In other words, an average child can first walk five steps unassisted at about 15 months of age. Does this mean that almost all children acquire this skill at an age of 15 months? Certainly not! An average is merely a sort of middle point. Half of all children will learn to walk five steps before 15 months; the other half will not acquire this talent until after 15 months. So, if a child is a month "late" in learning to walk, there is no need to panic. He has plenty of time.

From another perspective this same principle can be applied to adults. Some are talented at some things, others have other talents. Jane may be a better driver than Joan; Joan may be better at working with figures than Jane; Sue may be a better cook than either Jane or Joan. Yet they are all probably considered "normal."

In this respect, children are very much the same as adults; no two are the same. Because the basic equipment he is born with and because of the

4

unique experiences he has, one child has a pattern of individual strengths and weaknesses which no other child has. Some children are overall faster learners than others, some excel in athletics, some are more artistic, some become better readers than others—what psychologists call "individual differences." These differences between individuals are what makes life interesting. Imagine how dull the world would be if everyone were "average," if everyone had exactly the same abilities and interests.

The point of the story is that most of the time, individual differences in development are nothing to worry about. Only when they are extreme do they become cause for concern. Subsequent sections of this chapter will help determine just what is "extreme" when it comes to such individual differences.

Professionals usually talk about individual differences in various kinds of abilities in terms of a distribution called the *normal curve.* The normal curve is useful when we want to describe how a particular trait is distributed within a population. For example, if we were able to accurately meausre the intelligence of all the people in the United States we would end up with a normal curve depicting the distribution found. We could then sum all the scores and divide by the number of people we measured and get a mean or average. We could then compute a standard deviation of all the scores. The standard deviation for all the scores is used to indicate how many scores will be found under each part of the curve.

A standard deviation is a mathematical measure of the amount of variability occurring in a distribution curve. It is computed by a mathematical formula which defines one standard deviation above and below the mean as encompassing 68% of the population and two standard deviations above and below the mean as encompassing 96% of the population. The remaining 4% will show about 2% falling two standard deviations below and 2% above two standard deviations. Figure 1-1 depicts a normal curve for intelligence test scores together with a standard deviation and a percentage representation of the number of scores appearing under each area of the curve. For intelligence, the mean is 100 and the standard deviation is 15. We can see from the figure that very few people would attain scores below 55 or above 145 in our population.

The important thing to remember about the normal curve is that it provides a picture of the way many traits are distributed throughout the world. Although we used intelligence as our example, there are normal curve representations for height, weight, and many other physical and mental traits.

What happens on discovering that there is a real problem, that a child is delayed in some aspect of his or her development? Responses to problems such as this take many directions. First, there could be self-blame for being such a rotten parent. "Why else would Johnny develop this problem: I must not be doing a very good job!" It is natural to blame oneself for a child's problem. It is even natural to feel guilty. However, most of

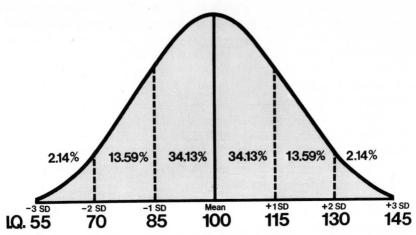

Figure 1-1 Normal distribution of intelligence test scores.

the time it simply is not true that it is all the parents' fault. Child-rearing is a complicated, demanding job: no one does it perfectly, and a child's problem may be due to something beyond parental control. Also, blaming oneself does not really help, it merely makes one feel worse. A parent may be embarrassed to admit the problem and ask for help—embarrassed to the point of inability to do so. We hope the parents' response will be closer to the second extreme which is taking some kind of constructive action to remedy the problem. It is good to acknowledge feelings of guilt or inadequacy, and talk about them, but not to the point of being so overwhelmed by guilt that one will not seek help.

A parent's response to discovering that his or her child has a problem is important enough to merit further discussion. Typically, when parents learn that their child is handicapped or delayed, they go through a grieving process, almost as if they had lost someone they love. This is to be expected, for in a sense they have lost something: their healthy, normal child. This grieving has five distinct stages.

Upon first being told that there is a problem, parents usually convince themselves that the problem does not exist: this stage is called denial. "No, not us! Surely our child can't be abnormal. The doctors must be wrong. There's nothing wrong with little Johnny!" It is almost as if something deep inside a parent is saying, "If I deny and ignore the problem, it will go away." This type of denial helps cushion the emotional blow.

Eventually, parents come to accept the fact that there is a problem, and they ask themselves, "Why me?" They become angry that their child has a problem, while a neighbor's children are normal. This stage is one of rage and anger. Following this, a stage called "bargaining" takes place. Parents in this stage look for others to make bargains with: "If I do this, Johnny will be OK." The bargains may be with anyone: doctors, psychologists, the child, even God.

Following the bargaining phase is a stage of depression. Parents feel that they have lost something, and that it is hopeless to try to get it back. They mourn the loss. After the depression runs its course, the final acceptance occurs. Parents accept the reality of the problem, and attempt to deal with it realistically.

Some might think it would be better if this long, painful grieving process could be avoided altogether. This is not true. It is a helpful healing mechanism for the parent's emotional life. Both parent and child will benefit in the long run if the process is allowed to run its natural course. Sometimes talking to trusted family or friends, or to a professional counselor, can help; but the feelings of each step must be experienced in order to reach a satisfactory resolution.

What is Development?

We have been talking about the parent. Now we will turn our attention to the child. In talking about a "normal" child, it was implied that a normal child is one whose development does not deviate markedly from developmental norms. But we have not explicitly defined what is meant by development. For our purpose, it can be called a process of change that a child undergoes en route to adult maturity.

Development proceeds as a child intereacts with his environment. A child is born with certain raw materials. As he interacts with his world and with individuals in that world, he practices using those materials and he becomes increasingly proficient in their use. In other words, he learns. Because development and learning depend on this interaction, they are affected by both raw materials (heredity) and experiences (environment) which are intertwined and interdependent. Trying to decide which is more important can be likened to arguing about whether the composer or the performer contributes more to a great musical performance.

During the course of development, a child is continually building upon his past experience. He actively seeks new experiences; he then integrates these new experiences with what he already knows. In the beginning he lives quite simply. He analyzes his environment in very gross, global ways, and his responses to it are equally gross and global. With time, he learns to make increasingly fine distinctions between the signals coming from his senses, and his repertoire of behaviors grows. This is called *differentiation*. For example, consider the process of becoming an expert on fine cooking. In the beginning it is difficult to tell the difference between foods of similar taste and most of what is cooked tastes about the same. Later on, it is possible to distinguish between tastes that are more and more alike. When preparing food, one must learn exactly when to add the right amount of the right seasoning. Child development proceeds in much the same way, as the child's world becomes increasingly differentiated.

Because no two children have exactly the same genetic equipment, and because no two children will be exposed to exactly the same influences, development might be expected to be a random sort of phenomenon, impossible to study or classify. However, although no two children will develop in exactly the same way, there will be similarities. In fact, child development seems to follow certain patterns, which can be recognized if one knows what to look for. When discussing how parents respond to learning that their child has a problem, we noted five stages in the typical parental response pattern. Just as grief seems to proceed in stages, child development proceeds in identifiable stages. Something in the genetic code that children carry seems to make them behave in certain ways at certain ages and makes them "blossom" in certain ways at certain times.

The notion of stages is common in child-rearing folklore. For example, almost any mother will talk about the "terrible twos." Also, consider the way in which children's social interactions change when they reach adolescence. And surely, most of us have heard the phrase, "He'll grow out of it." The advantages of child psychology over folklore is that it studies stages more systematically.

Thinking back to childhood, everybody may find some evidence of going through developmental stages, although they might not be thought of in those terms. Most of us remember almost nothing about our infancy, and very little about our preschool years. This memory gap cannot be explained by the passing of time alone; we did not remember these years very well when we were school-age children. Why? Long-term memory is not well developed in early years; thus early experiences were never stored in a form that we would recognize now. One may also remember a change in the way the world appeared around age 12 (give or take a little—remember individual differences?). Before that time, the world had a magical storybook quality. Afterward, nothing seemed the same; the magical quality was gone forever. Logical thought replaced the old magical way of apprehending the world. For example, knowing what road one was on while on an automobile trip seemed to take some of the beauty out of the scenery. Why? Because a new stage of mental development was entered around that time.

Different stages of development have different characteristics. They are "qualitatively," not "quantitatively" different. That is, they are not more or less, better or worse; they are just different. A very young child does not realize that people and objects still exist when he cannot see them, while an older child knows that "out of sight" does not mean "out of mind." Can anyone who has experienced the joy of playing peek-a-boo with a young child believe that this stage is inferior?

Often children cannot learn certain things until they have reached certain stages of development. For example, toilet training does not proceed smoothly until a child's nervous system has developed to a certain point. As another example, a typical child will not learn to think through several solutions to a problem until he nears pubescence. The parent must walk a fine line. On the one hand, the child needs training. On the other hand, care must be taken not to force him into attempting tasks he is incapable of; this could be very frustrating for him. Who ever said being a parent was easy?

Most children pass through developmental stages in the same sequence, however there are differences in the rates at which different children pass through them. All children learn to crawl before they learn to walk, but some children take longer than others to go from the crawling phase to the walking phase.

Development is a process that involves the whole child. Children are developing mentally, physically, and emotionally all at once; they do not develop mentally this week, physically next week, and emotionally the week after next. In addition, the different types of development all affect each other: a child's physical development affects his social development, his social development affects his emotional development, and so on. But if we tried to talk about all types of development at once, the results would be a hopeless muddle. So for convenience we will divide development into areas, and talk about each area separately. They are physical, motor, self-help, perceptual, language, mental, and social-emotional development. It must be kept in mind that the child is developing in other ways at the same time, and that there is nothing sacred about our developmental areas.

This chapter has discussed developmental norms and what development and stages are all about.

Under each area of development discussed in subsequent chapters are tips for fostering optimal development. These suggestions can make a bright child brighter, a good child better, a strong child stronger, an average child brighter, better, stronger, or a below-average child closer to the average. However, when there really is a problem, there is no substitute for competent professional help.

2 Physical Development

One of the most researched areas in development is motor development. We can document milestones in motor development even before birth. After the egg is fertilized it receives nurture from surrounding tissues and starts to grow. This growth is spectacular, since the organism is only about the size of a dot when prenatal development starts. From this small beginning, cells separate into layers and development proceeds rapidly. We use the term maturation to describe the changes which occur in structural development. A time line of prenatal development would appear as in Figure 2-1.

Once the child is born, he learns about his environment by the sensations he receives and by the movements he makes in response to these new sensations. The roles of sensation and movement are so closely related that a problem in either area would greatly hinder a child's early development. A child learns by taking an active role in exploring his environment and should be encouraged to do so by his parents.

Some patterns of development have been identified and are useful to anyone observing a young child.

1. Children develop in a sequential manner. This means that a parent need not worry if his child does not walk when he is a year old just because a particular chart says he should. Each new skill an infant acquires is based on other skills mastered earlier.

2. All skills seem to overlap. A child practices many activities at a time. Although he may seem to be at the "crawling stage," he can be seen to be attempting some basic standing and walking skills also.

3. A child's movements tend to be gross and general at first and then become more finely coordinated. This can be seen when an infant first attempts to reach out to grasp an object. It begins as a hit-and-miss operation, but after a few months of practice the infant can pick up the tiniest speck of dirt and deposit it neatly in his mouth.

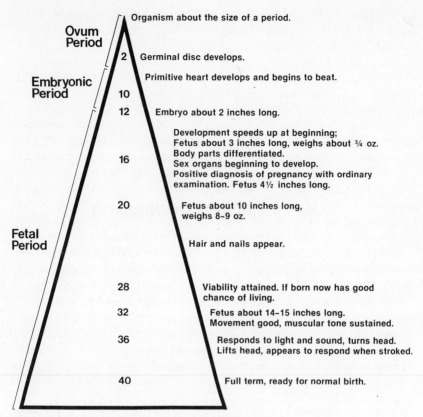

Ovum Period

Organism about the size of a period.

2   Germinal disc develops.

Embryonic Period

Primitive heart develops and begins to beat.

10

12   Embryo about 2 inches long.

Development speeds up at beginning;
Fetus about 3 inches long, weighs about ¾ oz.
Body parts differentiated.
16   Sex organs beginning to develop.
Positive diagnosis of pregnancy with ordinary
examination. Fetus 4½ inches long.

20   Fetus about 10 inches long,
weighs 8-9 oz.

Fetal Period

Hair and nails appear.

28   Viability attained. If born now has good
chance of living.

32   Fetus about 14-15 inches long.
Movement good, muscular tone sustained.

36   Responds to light and sound, turns head.
Lifts head, appears to respond when stroked.

40   Full term, ready for normal birth.

Figure 2-1 Time line of prenatal development.

4. Development progresses in a cephalocaudal or head to foot direction. This means that if we watched an infant, we would see development starting with the early moving of his head, the fixing of his gaze, and eye-hand coordination (Figure 2-2). All of these actions involve the upper part of the body. Actions involving the lower portions of the body such as sitting, crawling, and walking occur later.

5. Development progresses in a proximal-to-distal or "near-to-far" direction. For our purposes this means that the first areas of the body that a child learns to control are those close to his trunk. For example, a child

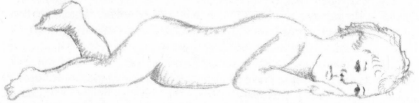

Figure 2-2 Development of an infant may start with a fixing of his gaze.

learns to coordinate his shoulders and elbows before he can use his wrists and hands. He uses his upper arm before his forearm, and his forearm before his hands and fingers.

It is more helpful to know these five patterns than to memorize a chart that tells "at what month a child does what." A parent can make up all sorts of activities based on these five ideas and thereby enhance the child's motor development.

If we do look at an infant's motor development, we can see many patterns developing. The newborn is a little bundle of flesh, still retaining qualities of his fetal position. His muscle tone tends to keep him in this position with most of his joints in a flexed or bent pattern (Figure 2-3). Over the next few months his greatest accomplishment will be to overcome gravity and to slowly develop enough extension of his body so that he can stand up. This can be observed in most of his efforts to move, beginning simply with his first attempts to lift his head while lying on his tummy, then pushing up onto his forearms, then up into a crawling position, and finally to standing.

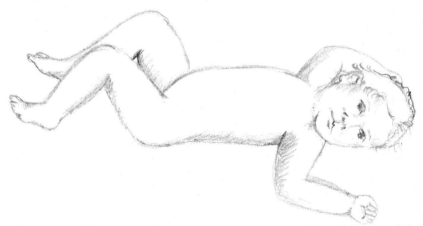

Figure 2-3 The newborn retains qualities of his fetal position, with most of his joints in a flexed or bent pattern.

This is a slow, continuous effort, coursing through the first year or so of an infant's life. Many of the changes in his motor development are molded by various reflexes. The infant's developing nervous system guides many of his ventures to take control of his movements through the fading in and out of a whole array of reflexes.

Many books have been written about early motor development on a month-by-month basis. A brief description of major accomplishments made during a child's first year of life will be followed by leaps and jumps through the child's gains made during the next three years.

0 to 3 Months

As mentioned earlier, an infant's limbs are held mainly in a flexed or bent position at birth and one of his major goals is to overcome gravity. Many of his early movements may appear random and disorganized; however, he is just getting his body ready for more skilled movements.

At birth, an infant who is placed on his tummy will be able to lift his head momentarily to turn it to the side. This is a protective mechanism so that he will not smother if he is accidently placed with his face down. By the time he is two months old, he can usually lift and hold his head up to look around for a few seconds while on his tummy. He begins to extend his neck and upper back and is gaining head control.

While lying on his back, the baby usually turns his head to one side and is not able to hold it so that he looks up. While lying with his head turned to one side, the arm toward which he is looking may tend to be straight with the opposite arm bent as in Figure 2-4. This is a reflex pattern commonly seen in infants and may be the beginning of the development of eye-hand coordination as the child begins to watch his hand and fingers move. Slowly, he will be able to hold his head with the face up and to follow people and objects with his eyes.

Although most infants do not learn to roll over during the first three months, there is another reflex that can be observed. If the baby's head is quickly turned all the way to one side while he is lying on his back, his whole body will follow and roll to the side or all the way onto the stomach. This is called the neck-righting reaction. When the baby begins to roll over on his own, he will no longer roll like a log, but will first turn his head, then his shoulders, and finally his hips and legs.

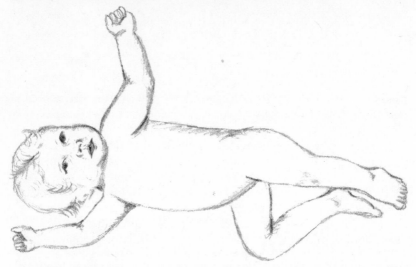

Figure 2-4 Eye-hand coordination begins with the infant gazing at the movement of his hands and fingers.

3 to 6 Months

Now the infant's movements appear to be more controlled and purposeful. While on his stomach, he is able to hold his head up for longer periods and begins to put weight on his arms while he looks around (Figure 2-5). We can see his development proceeding in the head-to-foot manner mentioned earlier in this chapter. He is gaining control of his shoulders and will soon be able to shift his weight from side-to-side in this position.

While lying on his back, the infant will be able to hold his head face up and begin to bring his hands together. He may put his fists in his mouth and grab at his clothing. Many infants may stare at their fingers for long periods. This seemingly insignificant feat is actually quite an accomplishment in comparison with the random, uncontrolled movements seen only a few months earlier.

Toward the end of the first six months, the child will reach for and crudely grasp rattles or toys offered to him. While on his stomach he may make a few successful attempts to support himself on one elbow while reaching out to grasp at a small toy in front of him. These hand movements will continue to become more and more refined.

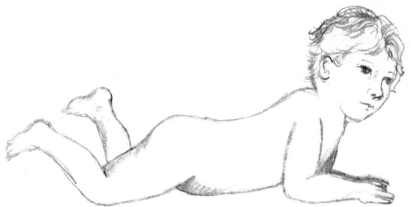

Figure 2-5 At 3 to 6 months, the infant may be able to put weight on his arms while he looks around.

6 to 9 Months

The next big step to be accomplished is the art of sitting. After being placed in a sitting position, the infant can first sit with his hands planted firmly on the floor as in Figure 2-6. Unfortunately, a strong wind can blow him over at first and he will make no attempt to catch himself. Although his head control is quite good, his sitting balance, which requires the control of his trunk muscles, is not yet well developed. Soon he will be able to sit using only one hand for balance, then unsteadily without the use of his hands. By the end of this period, the baby will be able to sit unassisted, reach for toys many inches away, and begin to twist and turn while sitting, rarely losing his balance. Quite an astounding feat!

Rolling activities are now more controlled and many infants roll all around the house as a very effective means of locomotion. The rolling motion has become more segmental, with the head or legs initiating the movement and then the rest of the body following, part-by-part. The child can stop the rotation at any point and hold the position in order to look at something or to reach for a toy.

Another skill which is usually begun later during this period is crawling on hands and knees. This skill varies greatly from child to child. As an infant becomes older, he becomes more of an individual and although many reflex patterns continue to guide his motor development, he has the final say-so in most instances. More specifically, one child may go from creeping on his stomach to crawling on hands and knees, and then to standing and walking. Another child may get around by rolling everywhere, then by crawling for a short time and then walking. Still another child may never or almost never crawl and just begin walking. Often this child, after he has learned to walk, may begin to crawl more, especially when playing on the floor. It is usually more efficient to crawl a few feet to retrieve a toy than to stand up, walk two steps, and then sit down again.

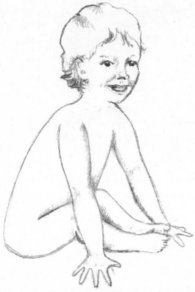

Figure 2-6   From 6 to 9 months the infant may be able to sit up.

9 to 12 Months

Although some children walk before they are a year old, most get around by crawling during this period. They continue to perfect this skill, strengthening their proximal muscles, that is, the ones at the shoulders and hips. In the normal crawling pattern, often called reciprocal crawling, one arm and the opposite leg are moved at the same time. This reciprocal pattern lays a basis for a normal walking pattern in which the arms swing opposite to the movement of the legs.

In general, as a child develops various motor skills, he can usually maintain a position before he can assume it. For example, a child can sit before he can get into a sitting position; he can stand holding onto a couch before he can pull himself up into this position. Another noticeable pattern is that usually a child first will be able to hold a position rigidly as if hanging on for dear life, and then with practice will be able to relax and control himself more. At first, a child will stand stiffly hanging onto the couch. Soon he will begin to shift his weight a little from side to side as he moves his head to look around. Then he may begin to reach out for a toy and even start to take a step or two to the side and so a child learns to stand and walk.

Finger and hand skills are developing rapidly too. The once crude grasp now becomes more of a pinching motion, first with the thumb and next two fingers, and then with the thumb and index finger only (Figure 2-7). The child can control the opening and closing of his hands to a greater degree. While only a few months ago his fingers had to be pried loose when he accidently grabbed his mother's hair, the baby can now willfully let go—if he wants to!

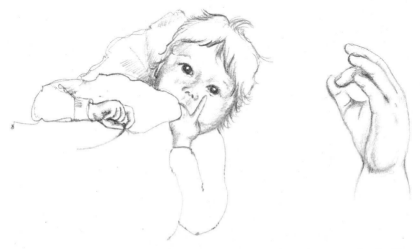

Figure 2-7   Finger and hand skills develop. The grasp becomes more of a pinching motion.

12 to 18 Months

Most children learn to walk during this period. Usually, Mom and Dad have been coaxing their child along and giving him plenty of opportunity to practice. After hanging onto the couch for the last few months, the one-year-old one day will take a step or two unassisted. Slowly he will perfect his walking over the next year or two. At first, the feet are kept wide apart to give the baby a broader base of support. His arms are held up high to aid balance further. He does not develop the reciprocal movement of his arms and legs until he is two to three years old.

Some of the fine motor tasks which the child accomplishes include stacking two blocks, scribbling on a paper when shown how, putting a raisin or other small object into a narrow-mouthed container, and dumping a block out of a cup. These skills incorporate cognitive or intellectual concepts with motor tasks. The child must be ready intellectually, as well as physically, when learning to imitate simple tasks.

18 to 36 Months

Walking skills continue to improve. The child can start and stop walking more accurately; he can turn sharper corners, walk sideways, and backwards, and even on his tiptoes. He learns to go up and down stairs, first on his hands and knees, then standing and using a handrail while putting two feet on each step. By the time he is three, a child can usually walk up and down stairs without holding on and by putting one foot on each step. He can also tap a ball in front of him with his toe at around two years, but will not be able to stand on one foot for a second or two until he is three or three and a half.

Building towers of blocks becomes a beguiling way to pass the time, first three blocks, then five, eight, and so on. By two, a child can usually turn the pages of a book one at a time and can put large beads on a string by the time he is two and a half.

36 to 48 Months

Between three and four a child learns a variety of skills. He learns to pedal a tricycle, he learns to walk a straight line, he learns to jump off a small step with both feet. All of these skills require increasing coordination. The child who used to move everything at once just to grasp a rattle can now perform intricate skills that require him to move only one part of his body while keeping the rest of his body still. In order for a child to be able to learn to cut with scissors or copy a straight line on paper, he must be able to hold and support the rest of his body.

During the first years of life, the child learns a multitude of motor skills. The motor developmental chart (Table 2-1) gives a series of motor skills which children learn during the first five years of life. Try to keep in mind the five principles of motor development which we discussed earlier in this chapter—skills developing in sequence, overlapping, moving from gross to fine, from head to foot, and from near the trunk to the extremities. By applying these principles all through a child's early years, his motor development can be enhanced greatly.

Table 2-1
Motor Developmental Chart

Gross Motor Skills	Fine Motor Skills
0 to 6 Months	
Raises his head off the floor for one second while on his stomach.	Turns his head from side to side to follow a toy.
Holds his head up for five seconds while on his stomach on the floor.	Moves his eyes across the midline.
Rolls from his side to his back.	Looks at his own hands for three seconds.
Holds his head steady when supported in a sitting position.	Grasps a toy when touched on his fingers.
Lifts his head and chest up for five seconds.	Reaches for an object.
Rolls from his back to his side.	Rakes and attains a bead.
Holds his head steady when pulled to a sitting position.	Picks up and holds two small blocks.
Rolls from his right to his left and back again.	
Assumes and maintains himself in a crawling position on his elbows.	
Rolls from his stomach to his back.	
Sits on the floor, leaning on his hands for one minute, with assistance.	
7 to 12 Months	
Lifts his head for five seconds while on back on the floor.	Transfers a block from one hand to the other.
Maintains himself on his stomach with his elbows straight and his legs straight behind.	Removes a small block from a cup.
Sits alone leaning on straight arms for 30 seconds.	Hits two blocks together.
Stands bearing his weight on his legs for 10 seconds with assistance at his waist.	Claps his hands together.
Crawls on his elbows for two feet.	Picks up a pellet with his thumb and forefinger.
Assumes and maintains a creeping position on his hands and knees.	Flings a ball without direction.
Moves from a creeping position to a sitting position.	Releases a small block into a cup.
	Releases a toy on command.

Table 2-1 *(continued)*

Sits erect for 30 seconds.
Stands holding onto a support for
 30 seconds.
Creeps on his hands and knees for
 two feet.
Pulls himself up to his knees.
Sits erect and reaches for a toy without
 using his hands for balance.
Pulls himself up to stand at a station-
 ary object.
Stands without hand held for 30 seconds.
Cruises around furniture to the right
 and left for at least five steps.
Walks with aid at his hips for at least
 ten steps.
Walks with one hand held for at least
 ten steps.

13 to 18 Months

Stands alone for at least three seconds.
Takes five steps alone.
Creeps backward down five steps.
Creeps up five steps.
Stoops to pick up a toy off the floor
 and stands up.
Walks up five steps with one hand held
 and one hand on the handrail.
Takes five steps backward.

Builds a tower of two blocks.
Draws a scribble on paper when shown
 how.
Puts a pellet into a bottle.
Dumps a block from a cup.
Builds a tower of three blocks.
Fills a cup with blocks.

19 to 24 Months

Walks down five steps with one hand
 held and one hand on the handrail.
Walks up five steps holding the handrail with one hand.
Runs ten steps.
Walks down five steps holding the
 handrail with one hand.

Builds a tower of five blocks.
Turns the pages of a book one at a
 time.
Taps a ball with toe.
Draws a vertical line when shown how.
Aligns two blocks (makes a train) when
 shown how.
Turns a doorknob to open a door.
Throws a small ball overhand.

25 to 36 Months

Walks on his tiptoes for five steps.
Jumps in place with both feet.
Stands on one leg with assistance.
Walks between two parallel lines which
 are eight inches apart, for five feet.
Leap-jumps from 18 inches.
Walks up five steps holding a hand-
 rail with one hand and alternating
 his feet.

Draws a circle when shown how.
Builds a tower of eight blocks.
Strings three large beads.
Draws a horizontal line when shown
 how.
Catches a large ball with arms straight.
Imitates a bridge.
Cuts a paper six inches with scissors.
Pours from a pitcher.

Table 2-1 *(continued)*

Rides a tricycle using the pedals.
Walks a straight line (one-inch width)
    for ten feet.
Jumps off a nine-inch platform with
    both feet.

37 to 48 Months

Stands on one leg for one second.   Draws a cross when shown how.
Walks five feet on a four inch balance   Copies a circle.
    beam.
Step-hops for five feet (skips lame-
    duck fashion).
Stands on one leg for five seconds.
Jumps down 28 inches with feet together.
Broad jumps nine inches.
Hops five times with assistance.

49 to 60 Months

Hops forward five times.   Draws a square when shown how.
Skips at least ten feet.   Draws a right descending diagonal
        when shown how.
    Draws a left descending diagonal when
        shown how.

Adapted with permission from: G. Casto, (Ed.). A Curriculum and Monitoring System. Logan, Utah: Utah State University Press, 1976.

3　Intellectual Development

Certainly one of the most basic and yet most misunderstood factors in human development is intelligence. Intelligence is intimately related to both learning and language and in general seems to encompass the kinds of skills needed to cope with all sorts of problem-solving situations. Scientists have always been interested in the concept of intelligence, but their research efforts have not always borne fruit. Charles Darwin was the first to take a serious interest in intelligence, and he kept a series of baby biographies in an attempt to measure a child's intellectual development as reflected in behavior. Later Albert Binet, a French physician, who is generally recognized as the father of intelligence testing as we know it, focused on measuring the child's mental development by means of an exhaustive series of tasks performed.

Since Binet's time, a wide variety of people have attempted to develop tests that assess intelligence. His original definition has had a marked impact on test construction and on ways we try to describe intelligence. He originally felt that intelligence was the individual's capacity to think abstractly and to use abstract symbols. If we keep in mind that Binet developed his test in an educational setting and wanted to make educational predictions from the results of the test, it is easy to see why he emphasized verbal skills in his definition. In fact, a good point to remember is that intelligence tests in general predict success in academic endeavors. That is, they do not assess characteristics such as motivation, they do not assess some of the kinds of skills we think of as being creative, and they do not assess many of the kinds of attributes seen as being necessary for success in life. What they do measure with a fair degree of accuracy is the ability of a child to succeed in academic or educational settings.

A few points to keep in mind about intelligence tests is that they are in no way a measure of a child's inherited ability, they are heavily weighted with verbal abstract skills, and they assess different abilities at different age levels. For example at year two, intelligence tests contain many items related to language and motor development; at year five they begin to include verbal skills; and by year thirteen, they are heavily loaded with verbal comprehension and reasoning. We must also remember that intelligence tests are culture-bound. This means that it is extremely difficult, if not impossible, to develop tests which assess subjects uniformly across cultures. Within each nation, tests are usually geared to the dominant culture. This means in the United States that if the child taking the test is not American-born, does not speak English, and has not been exposed to a white middle-class culture, he is penalized. A great deal of controversy has arisen over this point. Many people feel that we should do away with intelligence tests since they do discriminate against minority groups. Again, it is useful to remember the point we began with that intelligence tests are valid only for making predictions about school success. Since they do this job well, we can only conclude that it is the culture that is discriminatory and not the tests.

Jean Piaget has perhaps done more than any other scientist to chart the development of intelligence in infancy. His theory of intellectual development terms the period from birth to two years of age as the *sensorimotor stage,* the period from two to seven the *preoperational stage,* the period from seven to eleven years the *concrete operations stage,* and the period from eleven on as the *formal operations stage.*

In the sensorimotor stage, the reflexes which an infant possesses at birth are organized behavior patterns which enable him to interact with his environment. These simple patterns of behavior, which he calls "schemas," become linked with other patterns of behavior and become coordinated and generalized. As the infant gains experience, he tends to repeat behaviors that produce certain results. Subsequently the infant directs behavior toward objects and events in his environment and begins to develop a sense of cause and effect relationships. If you have ever watched a baby with a rattle, you may have noted that, as part of his experimentation, he will let the rattle drop on purpose sometimes. His interest now is not only on the rattle, but what can happen to it based upon his actions.

At this time also, the child acquires the concept of object permanence. Development of this concept provides the basis for a new level of reasoning, one in which problems may be solved through mental operations and not just through physical activity.

When a child enters the preoperational stage, he is increasingly able to deal with his environment in an abstract manner. He begins to be able to visualize solutions to problems and no longer uses a strictly trial and error approach. The child is also able to imitate others and uses this skill to solve problems.

Two important characteristics of this preoperational stage are that 1) the child's immediate perceptions dominate his problem-solving efforts, and 2) the child's thinking and his point of view are centered about himself. As an example, if a child knows that two portions of a substance are equal in size and they are subsequently formed in such a way that they do not look equal, his immediate perception will dominate and he will insist that one is longer or taller.

The concrete operations stage of thinking is characterized by the increasingly logical nature of the child's thought. He learns the principles of conservation and no longer lets his immediate perceptions dominate. In addition, he begins to understand the operations involved in number concepts and how objects can be classified into larger, broader, and more general categories. Finally, during this period, he loses his egocentric reasoning patterns and begins to consider the points of view of those around him.

As the child enters adolescence, he acquires the ability to think in abstract terms, to manipulate abstract symbols, and to solve problems and to reason in an abstract manner. Piaget calls this period the formal operations stage.

For Piaget, intelligence emerges as a consequence of experience and maturation. He believes that intelligence involves a progressively organized adaptation to the environment and that both maturation and experience play key roles. Others have looked at the development of intelligence differently. Arthur Jensen has stated that intelligence is largely determined by heredity, and others have stated that it is largely determined by the environment in which one grows up.

Certainly, the old saying that "one should choose one's parents wisely" testifies to the heritability of intelligence behaviors. At the same time, it is clear that the environment from conception on plays a major role in shaping intelligence. Scientists are currently studying the interaction between heredity and environment. It is obvious that the argument will continue.

In stimulating intellectual development, people have drawn heavily on Piaget's conception of development. Sensorimotor development is stimulated by providing grasping, visual tracking, and imitative activities. The table below depicts Piaget's stages and suggests behaviors that may be elicited at each stage.

Table 3-1
Piaget's Stages of Intellectual Development

Stage and Approximate Age	Characteristic Behavior
I. Sensorimotor Operations	
1. Reflexive (0 to 1 month)	Simple reflex activity; example: kicking.
2. Primary Circular Reactions	
(1 to 4½ months)	Reflexive behavior becomes elaborated and coordinated; example: eye follows hand movements.

Table 3-1 *(continued)*

3. Secondary Circular Reactions (4½ to 9 months)	Repeats chance actions to reproduce an interesting change or effect; example: kicks crib, doll shakes, so kicks crib again.
4. Coordination of Secondary Schema (9 to 12 months)	Acts become clearly intentional; example: reaches behind cushion for ball.
5. Tertiary Circular Reactions (12 to 18 months)	Discovers new ways to obtain desired goal; example: pulls pillow nearer in order to get toy resting on it.
6. Invention of New Means through Mental Combinations (18 to 24 months)	Invents new ways and means; example: uses stick to reach desired object.
II. Preoperational	
1. Preconceptual (2 to 4 years)	Capable of verbal expression, but speech is repetitious; frequent egocentric monologues.
2. Intuitive (4 to 7 years)	Speech becomes socialized; reasoning is egocentric; "to the right" has one meaning—to child's right.
III. Concrete Operations (7 to 11 years)	Mobile and systematic thought organizes and classifies information; is capable of concrete problem-solving.
IV. Formal Operations (11 years upward)	Can think abstractly, formulate hypotheses, engage in deductive reasoning, and check solutions.

Adapted from: W.B. Stephens and J.A. McLaughlin. Analysis of performances by normals and retardates on Piagetian reasoning assessments. *Percept Mot Skills,* 1971.

4   Language Development

Only recently have we begun to tease out and answer some of the questions regarding language development in children. We have started now to describe some of the normative stages through which the child proceeds in language development. Contrary to supposition, the infant does have other sounds in his repertoire in addition to crying. Although crying is what most parents hear for the first few weeks of a baby's life, the child has other vocalizations at his command. Crying is important to the young infant because it is his primary communication system. With crying and the few motor movements the child possesses, he responds to stimuli such as hunger, fatigue, or discomfort. Lest we forget, it might be important to emphasize that throughout cultures crying is one of the most powerful communicative devices known.

When parents stand over a crib and hear their baby first make a cooing sound they usually associate this with the beginnings of language. This is not true. Cooing is a somewhat innate response occurring at a particular stage of development, and it lacks the flexible structure of language. The infant coos whenever he feels like it, not in response to something. Cooing usually begins to disappear at about eight weeks after birth.

In addition to crying, another important precursor to language is babbling. When the child is about six months old he begins to string together a great number and variety of sounds. Watching a child doing this one might think that he was experimenting with types of sounds, intonation, and even pitch. Nearly all babies will babble on their own but it has been demonstrated in several studies that if we attend to the babbling by smiling or fondling the infant, he will babble a great deal more than otherwise. As an infant matures, his babbling begins to resemble his parents' speech. We still do not completely understand why this is so. It may be because parents reinforce the babbling which in their perception is somewhat akin to language. On the other hand, maybe babbling is only a "warm-up" that allows the infant to understand how the sound he makes relates to the movement of his tongue or mouth. In this way it may contribute to his ability to produce speech rather than his ability to understand language. As Lennenburg demonstrated in 1964, there are infants who have never babbled or uttered any bit of language who yet understand new and complex sentences.

As early as the first ten days of his life, an infant may be able to sound four of the 35 basic *phonemes,* or sounds, that make up our language. The first sounds bear no relation to the sounds he hears about him. Babies throughout the world all pronounce the same phonemes as they progress through the stages of babbling. Later the child drops those sounds that are not required in speaking specific languages. Although we still do not understand completely why this is done, it is probable that imitation and the parents' selective attention to the sounds that make up (in our case) the English language cause the others to drop out. In the course of language development vowels outnumber consonants by about five to one in the infant's speech for the first four weeks. After that time, the use of vowels decline and consonants begin to predominate. At the age of six months most babies are capable of making almost all the vowel sounds but production of consonants increases even more rapidly. Soon after his first birthday, the infant is uttering more consonants than vowels as he approaches the adult ratio of one to four consonants for each vowel. As he grows older, the infant also makes more and more sounds in any given period of time. At eight weeks he averages 63 sounds and at 24 weeks his average rises to 74 sounds.

By age one year the child learns to distinguish vowels from consonants and begins combining them, which leads to rudimentary language forms. While there are vast differences in the ages at which infants first begin to speak, the average infant usually says his first word at about one year of age. From that first word the child's vocabulary develops by leaps and bounds. By the time he is four he will have approximately 1200 words in his vocabulary.

Once a child knows the meaning of a number of words, he comes to grips with syntax. Syntax in English consists largely of ordering words or putting words in the correct order in a sentence. Next, the child learns from the way words are used in sentences what class the words belong to so that they can be transformed and used in contexts other than those in which they were learned. Obviously the young child does not know the formal names of various word classes such as nouns and verbs, but once he understands syntax so that he can use a word's position and connected terms as clues, he can begin to make transformations. By age four or five most children know the proper transformation rules of English as in changing from singular to plural.

Children learn to combine words at 18 to 24 months. They begin with simple two-word phrases or "sentences" but by the time they are four or five they utter complex sentences and demonstrate mastery of our complex grammar.

Many individual differences in communicative skills, especially vocabulary, have been shown to exist between different groups of children. The sex of the child, his family size, his parents' occupations, educational level, the number of languages spoken in the home, and parental attitudes toward their children's speech are just a few of the factors associated with individual differences. Some presumed handicaps to adequate language development such as bilingualism are still not clearly understood and may have been greatly exaggerated in their influence. We do know that social class differences in language and in verbal facility are apparent early in life. Middle and upper class children are superior to lower class children in vocabulary, sentence structure, and articulation. The differences seem to be due to differences in the language environments of the different groups.

Language development also interacts with cognitive development. As the child's facility in language increases, his thinking and problem-solving skills increase also. Increasing language skills are also thought to pave the way for progress in complex learning activities.

Although milestones have been documented in the onset and development of speech, variability among children is substantial. Three major types of problems can be identified, however, which suggest that intervention is required. These include substantial language delay, articulation problems, and stuttering.

Many professionals are now emphasizing early identification and intervention for children whose speech is delayed. Developmental language programs are available which can accelerate the language development of a child whose speech is delayed. Children with significant language delays should therefore be referred to professionals as soon as possible.

Articulation problems involve errors in the production of speech sounds or phonemes. Articulation errors are common during the early phases of language development. After a child reaches school age, however, articulation errors require referral to a professional for assessment and remediation.

Stuttering is a familiar speech disorder but it is also a puzzling one. Defined as frequent interruptions of speech production by repetition or prolongation of sounds or syllables, stuttering commonly occurs in young children. If it persists or becomes severe, referral to a professional is again indicated. Approximately one to two percent of school-age children exhibit this problem.

Stimulating a child's language development can begin when the child is born. Holding the child and talking to him apparently has beneficial effects. Providing models for the child to imitate and using elaborated and expanded language systems when the child begins to utter words is also of significant benefit.

5 Sensory and Perceptual Development

Becoming aware of what is going on around us and within us are functions of sensation and perception. Figuring out what to do involves cognition, and acting upon it involves the motor component.

The first two of these processes, sensation and perception, are the subjects of this section. Scientifically, sensation and perception are quite different, as will be shown. So, it is important to stress the difference throughout this section. In practice, however, sensation and perception are interrelated.

SENSATION AND PERCEPTION

Sensation refers to the collection of raw data about the world around us and inside of us, and the relaying of this information from the sense organs (eyes, ears, etc) to the brain. If the process were to end here, we would be left with a mass of meaningless stimulation. We must make sense out of the information. This is where perception enters in. Perception refers to the internal process of converting meaningless stimulation into useful information.

In the visual sphere, sensation refers to seeing an object; perception refers to recognizing the object. Most of the time, sensation and perception occur so automatically that we are not aware that there are two things going on. For example, look at the number on this page. It can be recognized immediately, without awareness that in order to recognize it, the light waves reflecting off of it must reach the eyes and initiate nerve impulses to the brain, which must then take the information contained in those impulses, compare it with things which have been experienced in the past, and figure out that the design is a number, what the number is, and what the number means.

Most of us are born with a marvelous array of standard equipment which allows us to keep tabs on what is going on in the world around us. Much of this equipment is subsumed under the notion of the five senses: vision, hearing, smell, taste, and touch. Actually, touch is not one sensation, but is a combination of several sensations: light, touch, pressure, pain, warmth, and cold. In addition, there are senses which are vitally important to us, but which we usually do not think much about. For example, we are continually keeping track of how full our stomachs are, what positions our arms and legs are in, and whether we are right side up, upside down, or sideways. This type of sensation is so automatic that we are not really aware that it is happening. We would only notice it if we suddenly had to to without it.

Children are born with most of their senses in working order. Those that are not fully developed at birth generally develop quickly. Perception is another matter entirely. For the most part, children are not born with the ability to perceive—that is, to organize the information coming from their senses. In addition, perception does not seem to develop automatically as a child matures. On the contrary, it is a skill which must be learned through experience. A child only learns to make sense out of his world by living in it, manipulating it, and experiencing it.

An example will highlight the importance of experience in learning to perceive. A peculiar phenomenon occurs when people who have been blind all of their lives suddenly have their sight surgically restored. Their eyes work just the same as normal eyes; they see the same lights and patterns. However, their owners have had no experience using their eyes. So even though they can now see, they have not had enough experience seeing to be able to perceive visually. Learning to perceive visually is a slow, gradual process for them, much as it is for a child.

Now that it is established that perception is something that must be learned, it must be stressed that perceptual skill is an important prerequisite for other types of learning occurring later in life. On the surface, perception per se does not appear to be particularly important once a child reaches middle childhood. If he does not acquire adequate perceptual skills early in life, however, he will have difficulty mastering more complex mental tasks later on. Adequate performance in school will be much more difficult for him than for a child with a strong background in basic perceptual activities. For example, the ability to perceive forms correctly is a very important prerequisite for learning to read. In fact, psychologists are able to predict a child's first grade reading achievement by assessing how well he can perceive and copy geometric designs. It is important that a child be permitted and encouraged to manipulate his environment so that he can acquire the perceptual skills that are necessary for later mental development.

Sensory and perceptual development are two of the most important developmental tasks that the child must master between birth and 18 months of age. The first of these tasks involves coordinating sensory information. To the infant, each sense modality is a separate world. He does not realize that the baby rattle which he feels in his hand is the same baby rattle that he sees or hears. He is much like the formerly blind, newly-sighted adult who does not realize that the object he sees is the wooden block with which he is familiar through touch. By manipulating and experiencing objects in his world, the infant gradually learns that the feel of an object is analogous to the sight of it, which in turn is analogous to the sound the object makes. That is, he learns to make connections between his senses, to form a perceptual world as we know it.

The other major sensory-perceptual task of the child up to the age of 18 months is the development of object permanence. At first when an object disappears from sight, it may as well no longer exist. When the child coordinates information from his various senses, he begins to develop the notion that objects are concrete entities. Through repeated experiences with the same objects, he realizes that they are permanent and continue to exist even when they are no longer visible. Along with developing a sense that objects are permanent, the child develops a sense that he too is a permanent, concrete being, and that he is separate from other objects around him. The role of this discovery in personality development is discussed in the section on social-emotional development.

It has already been stated that a child's perceptual development occurs because he manipulates objects in his environment. This implies that the child is not passively bombarded with stimulation, but rather that he actively seeks certain kinds of experiences. Even at birth, the child's sensory and perceptual processes are active. This is sufficient background for proceeding to discussions of sensory and perceptual development in the various sense modalities. Sensory-perceptual development will be discussed in each sense modality separately, keeping in mind the developing interdependence of the various sense modalities as the child learns to coordinate the information from the different senses into unified perception.

VISUAL DEVELOPMENT

The infant is born with his visual system fairly well developed. He seems to react to differences in light intensity. He is able to focus on and follow a moving light. A newborn does not seem to be focusing his attention on anything in particular because there are a few ways in which his visual apparatus differs from that of the adult. The center of his retina (the area inside the back of the eyeball which records the image of what the person is looking at and relays the information toward the brain) is not fully developed. The muscles that adjust the thickness of the lens in the front of his eye are not yet fully operational, so the lens is large and spherical. His eyeball is shorter from front to back than that of the adult and the nerve fibers carrying visual images from the eyes to the brain are not completely insulated yet.

With such a vague, confusing visual world, one would expect that the infant would passively glance at anything that happens to be in his visual field. Surprisingly, this is not the case. He actively looks for certain kinds of visual stimulation, preferring to look at objects with complex patterns on them, rather than simple ones. He prefers objects with sharply defined black and white portions, and would rather look at a human face or a form resembling a face than at a nonhuman object.

The infant probably has rudimentary color vision at birth. His ability to tell the difference between different colors improves gradually from birth to three years of age. At the age of one year, the average child can discriminate between bright green, bright yellow, bright red, and bright blue. At this age, he seems to prefer red objects. By age three the color-discriminating ability of the average child is well developed.

The infant does not use both eyes together when he looks at something. Rather, for the first six to eight weeks of life, he fixates one eye on an object, and lets the other eye relax. As a result, he is not able to fixate on an object for any length of time, and probably does not perceive depth very accurately. He becomes able to fixate on an object for a sustained period of time at the age of four or five weeks.

To demonstrate why depth perception is difficult for the infant before he learns to coordinate his two eyes, a little experiment is helpful. First, close one eye. Then hold your right hand about two feet in front of your face, and point your right index finger to the left. Finally, with one eye still closed, hold out your left arm with your left index finger pointing to the right, and try to touch your right index finger with your left index finger. Chances are that you missed on your first attempt. Now try the same thing, but with both eyes open. It is a lot easier that way. Because the infant only fixates on objects with one eye, his depth perception is much like an adult's with one eye closed.

Before a child can learn to perceive depth accurately, the coordination of his eye muscles must develop to the point where his vision is "binocular," that is, where he uses both eyes together in a coordinated manner. In addition to requiring coordination of eye muscles, this process also requires that the nerve endings in the retina be fully developed. Most of this development occurs during the first year of life.

As the infant begins to progress beyond the stage of fixating with one eye while relaxing the other, he begins to look at objects by rapidly alternating between the use of one eye and the other. This usually begins in the sixth to eighth week of life. During this phase, the child will often look cross-eyed. Between the ages of four and six months the child gradually learns truly to coordinate his two eyes, so that they converge upon the object that he is looking at.

That six-month-old babies are able to use their two eyes to perceive depth is evident from research studies employing the "visual cliff." In these studies, a child is placed on a large plate of thick glass. Under half of this glass is a checkerboard pattern in contact with the glass. Under the other half, the checkerboard drops off to a depth of a couple of feet below the glass. The result is a "cliff" several feet deep, from which the child is in no danger of falling thanks to the glass. When a six-month-old child is placed on the glass, he typically refuses to crawl over to the deep side, even if his mother beckons him over to that side. This avoidance suggests that the child at this age is able to preceive depth.

It is of interest to note that children who are "later crawlers" are more likely to cross over to the deep side of the visual cliff. Apparently, they are somewhat slower at learning depth perception, which seems to develop concurrently with the ability to crawl. Once a child is able to move about in his environment, depth and the localization of objects in space become important to him. In addition, depth perception is important in using vision to direct one's hand in reaching for an object. This is another reason why depth perception develops around the time when the child is beginning to explore his environment actively.

The development of depth perception does not stop as soon as the child begins to crawl. Children continue to learn about spatial relationships in their world throughout their preschool years, and probably on into their school years. Early visual perceptual learning, however, is not limited to the development of depth perception. More important to visual perception is learning that involves the issues of *object constancy* and *object permanence.* The latter is one of the most important developmental tasks for the young child.

Before a child can develop a sense that objects are permanent, he must learn that the size and shape of an object are constant. Recognition of size constancy usually begins to develop around the age of 10 weeks. In some precocious children the skill may be fairly well developed by this age; however, the average child realizes at around six months of age that familiar objects do not change size. The child will still have trouble with unfamiliar objects and will have a tendency to confuse concepts such as "big," "medium," and "small," until six years of age. Size constancy reaches its adult level by age 10.

Another step toward the sense of object permanence is the achievement of shape constancy. Hold a dinner plate or some other round object at an angle and look at it. What shape is it? It is round even though the shape registered is oval. The true shape of the object can be recognized because at some point in childhood the notion of shape constancy has been developed and objects can be recognized regardless of their orientation in space. Most children learn to do this before age two.

So eventually children learn that objects have certain characteristics that do not change. Shape does not change despite changes in orientation, size does not change despite changes in distance, color does not change despite changes in lighting. Children also begin to notice that the same objects appear and reappear. Gradually, these kinds of experiences lead them to the belief that objects are permanent.

To the child less than five months of age, out of sight means out of mind. Objects cease to exist when they leave the visual field. Between five and eight months of age the child realizes that this is not the case and will look down for something dropped. If he cannot find the something, he will look were he last saw it. An eight- to 12-month-old child, will remove the cover that has been placed over an object to find it. Thus, he is beginning to acquire a sense that objects are located in space, that they are permanent, that there is more to the world than that which is immediately visible. He still fails to realize, however, that an object might not still be in the last place where he saw it. Between 12 and 18 months he begins to look in different places for an object, but he gives up quickly if he does not find it. By 18 months, the average child finally has developed internal images of objects, and thus truly knows that they are permanent. At this stage, children are fascinated by peek-a-boo, because this game violates their newfound notion of object permanence.

Object permanence helps change the child's world from one of disorder, unpredictability, and chaos to one of order and stability. It is also important in social-emotional development for "objects are permanent" means "people are permanent," which means "I am permanent," which means "I am separate from my environment."

Another perceptual task of early life involves learning to discriminate between different people. This is discussed in more detail in the section on social-emotional development.

Although the child's visual-perceptual world is fairly mature by the age of one or one and one-half years, some perceptual skills develop later. The preschool child knows that solid objects are permanent and unchanging, but he does not develop the same feel for substances such as fluids until around age seven. This is known as "conservation of amount."

As children grow older, they learn to recognize objects from fewer and fewer clues. A four-year-old must look at an object fairly carefully and notice many aspects of it in order to recognize it. An older child, on the other hand, is able to glance at an object, notice just a few of the attributes of the object, and recognize what the whole object is by mentally filling in the gaps.

The developmental milestones for visual, sensory, and perceptual development are summarized in Table 5-1. It will be noted that six months seems to be a crucial age, at which many aspects of visual development become fairly mature.

Table 5-1
Developmental Milestones in Visual Sensory and Perceptual Development

Age	Developmental Milestones
Infancy	Cannot adjust lens: cannot focus each eye.
	Muscles not fully developed: cannot converge two eyes on object.
	Retina not fully developed: lacks visual acuity.
	Sees light, movement, and pattern, but cannot focus, cannot fixate for sustained period of time.
	Uses one eye only: lacks depth perception.
6 to 8 weeks	Alternates looking with each eye: may appear cross-eyed.
4 months	Can focus each eye: can follw object in any direction.
6 months	Visual acuity almost as good as that of adults.
	Depth perception fairly well developed.
	Differentiates familiar person from stranger
	Recognizes size constancy for familiar objects.
12 months	Can discriminate saturated colors.
18 months	Object permanence.
2 years	Shape constancy.
3 years	Mature color discrimination.
7 years	Conservation of amount.
8 years	Few reversal errors.

6 Self-Help Development

In general, the process of self-help development can be viewed as a change from dependence to independence. At birth, the human infant is completely helpless and completely dependent upon adults for survival. Human infants also remain helpless longer than infants of other species of animals. By the time a person becomes a young adult, he is able to care for himself almost completely. In a sense, development is a process by which a child takes over more and more of the responsibilities for caring for himself. So all aspects of child development could be considered "self-help development." But when we refer to the term here, we mean those aspects of development in which a child learns to take care of his own physical needs.

At first, the infant's nutritional and eliminative needs must be attended to by his parents. Gradually, and much to the parents' relief, the child learns to feed himself and to control elimination. For obvious reasons, these types of learning are important to parents. Perhaps because of this importance professional and parental attitudes about feeding and toilet training have tended to follow fads. Unfortunately, they have seldom been based on good solid facts. One of the purposes of this section is to discuss some of these fads and dispel some myths about them.

FEEDING, WEANING, AND EATING

Should a baby be breast- or bottle-fed? This question has provoked passionate statements from proponents of both points of view. The recent trend in this area has been in favor of breast feeding. The "experts" who favor breast feeding claim that cow's milk and commercial formulas contain harmful products such as radioactive strontium 90. They fail to mention, however, that this substance is carefully monitored in both cow's milk and formulas and that it may also appear in breast milk. Breast-feeding proponents also claim that breast feeding is the only "natural" way to feed a baby; that failure to breast feed is a sign of a mother's emotional maladjustment and will cause a child to develop emotional problems. They neglect to mention that modern technology and convenience is not inherently bad; that personal preference does not necessarily mean emotional maladjustment; and that a child's emotional state depends on much more than simply whether or not he was breast-fed.

On the other hand, advocates of bottle feeding cite a multitude of harmful substances that may appear in breast milk. They neglect to note that if a mother is careful about the foods and other substances she ingests and if she carefully monitors her own health (with the help of a physician), she can be fairly certain of producing healthy milk. Bottle-feeding proponents also claim that breast feeding produces overly dependent children. They seem to overlook the fact that early dependency between infant and mother is the basis for healthy emotional development and for the ability to express mature love as an adult.

The lack of an advantage for either method is supported by scientific research. In general, it has been found that children who were breast-fed and children who were bottle-fed do not differ in terms of their behavior and personality adjustment later in life. Neither breast nor bottle feeding ensures adequate psychological adjustment. In addition, there is no clear nutritional advantage for one method over the other.

Although in general, breast and bottle feeding are about the same in terms of nutrition and psychological effects, it is important that each individual mother choose the feeding method with which she is most comfortable. The research studies mentioned have dealt with contact groups, comparing children who had already been either breast-fed or bottle-fed. For their own personal reasons, mothers of the children in the studies selected how they wanted to feed their babies. What the research findings really mean is not that any mother can use either feeding method successfully, but rather that as long as a mother does what is comfortable for her and her family, her child is unlikely to suffer ill effects. So, each mother must decide which method is best for herself. Regardless of which method is chosen, there are certain things one should know.

If a mother decides that she is most comfortable breast feeding her child, she must remember that the nutrients and calories in breast milk come from the food she eats. This means that she should eat a well-balanced diet which includes 800 to 1000 calories per day more than she ordinarily eats. She should be careful about taking medications during the period of breast feeding. In addition, Rh-negative babies are particularly sensitive to the harmful effects on the liver of a hormone that is sometimes found in breast milk. A physician should be consulted for specifics on these last two points. Finally, the effects that breast feeding might have on the mother and the rest of the family must be considered.

Bottle feeding has its own set of challenges. For one thing, bottle feeding is easier to "louse up" than breast feeding. Instructions that come with commercial formulas must be read and followed carefully. If there is something in the instructions that is not understood, ask someone! A pediatrician is a good resource.

Breast feeding serves two important functions in addition simply to providing a baby with nourishment: it brings the baby into intimate physical contact with the mother, and the mutual pleasure involved creates a strong emotional bond between mother and child. Both the physical contact and the emotional bond are crucial to the child's later emotional well-being. This does not mean that breast feeding is the only way to produce an emotionally stable child; rather, it means that bottle feeding should be performed in such a way that it approximates breast feeding. When an infant is being bottle-fed, he should be cradled as if he were being breast-fed. Propping the bottle in position for feeding should not be done on more than an occasional basis. One of the advantages of bottle feeding is that other family members can perform some of the feeding. This increases their involvement with the child, and takes some of the load off the mother. However, having the mother do the majority of feeding will facilitate the development of a healthy emotional bond between mother and child.

Research on feeding schedules indicates that when parents follow the type of schedule they are comfortable with, the child's physical and emotional health are not adversely affected regardless of the type of schedule chosen. If mother and family adapt well to demand feeding, fine. If the infant's feeding demands are running everybody ragged, it might be worthwhile to adjust his feeding schedule so that it places less stress on the family's lifestyle.

Opinion on the "best" way to wean a child is divided, even today. Many textbooks recommend that babies be weaned gradually: gradually introducing cup feeding while fading out the breast or bottle, and perhaps still allowing the child to have a bottle at bedtime. As the argument goes, a gradual change from sucking to drinking is less likely to "frustrate" the child than an abrupt change. However, one of the authors has recently spoken with a pediatrician who recommends the "cold turkey" method of weaning: simply taking away the breast or bottle and telling the child, "It's all gone!" This pediatrician also believes that a bottle at bedtime is unhealthy, because warm milk remains in the child's mouth all night and may cause tooth decay.

For the average child, weaning is begun in the second half of the first year of life. By the age of six months, most children are ready to try drinking milk from a cup (they are able to sit up and reach for a cup), and children at this age are beginning to want more mobility and control than breast or bottle feeding permits. In some special circumstances, weaning may be started earlier, but in most cases this is the optimal time.

To summarize, it seems that despite arguments to the contrary, it does not really matter how an infant is fed, or when, or how he is weaned, except in special circumstances. What is important is that the feeding practices chosen are ones that the mother is comfortable with in terms of what each practice will mean to family life. Feeding practices may indeed influence a child's personality, but the emotional climate in the family is important, too. Selecting feeding practices that the family likes can contribute to a healthy emotional environment for the infant.

Most children are born with the reflexes necessary to feed from a nipple. The newborn will turn his head from side to side when he is stimulated by a nipple touching his face. When he finds the nipple, he will open his mouth, close his lips on it and suck. After about one week, the random side-to-side head turning will give way to directed head turning: that is, when the infant feels the nipple touch his face, he will turn his head in the appropriate direction.

By the age of about four weeks, the child will be able to suck and swallow liquids from a spoon that is put to his mouth. He will develop the ability to swallow pureed or strained food between the ages of 13 weeks and seven months. By the age of six months, a child is usually able to bring his hand to his mouth. By eight to nine months of age he will begin to hold and play with a spoon. These last two skills are prerequisites for later eating behaviors.

By nine months of age, a child is able to hold the breast or bottle while feeding from it. At roughly the same age, the child will learn to drink from a cup or glass that is held for him. Toward the end of the first year, children develop the ability to reduce lumps in their food by chewing them. When this happens, they are ready to eat "infant solids" or lumpy "junior foods" from a spoon. Between the ages of 10 and 14 months, children learn to finger-feed themselves, and they are able to chew and swallow solid food.

Appetites during the first year of life tend to be rather voracious. However, around the age of one year, they usually show a marked decline. This change is due to changes in the child's physiology. Parents should be aware of this so they do not try to force their children to eat more than necessary.

Between the ages of 12 and 16 months children learn to hold a cup with both hands and drink from it. Around 15 months of age they begin to feed themselves with a spoon, although at this stage as much food ends up on the bib, table, and floor as in the mouth. By 18 months they are generally able to feed themselves with a spoon without spilling much. However, they may still prefer using their fingers beyond the age of two years.

Early in the second year of life, children typically begin to eat with a fork, although they hold the fork in their fists. Around the middle of the second year, they can learn to drink from a straw (with assistance) and toward the end of the second year, they learn to hold spoons and forks underhand instead of in their fists, and to sit in their chairs throughout meals. Around the end of the second year, children usually lean to unwrap foods such as candy and crackers in waxed paper.

During the third year of life, children learn to drink while holding a glass held in one hand, to use a napkin, and to clean up their own spills. They also learn to serve themselves from serving bowls. During year four, they learn to clear their place settings from the table after meals, to chew with their mouths closed, and to spread food with a knife. During year five, they learn to cut foods with a fork, to pass serving bowls, and to help in setting the table.

The development of eating behavior is summarized in Table 6-1.

Table 6-1
Developmental Milestones in Feeding and Eating

Age	Developmental Milestones
Birth	Random nipple-seeking; closes mouth on nipple, sucks, swallows.
1 week	Directed nipple-seeking.
4 weeks	Takes liquid offered by spoon.
13 to 28 weeks	Takes pureed or strained foods from spoon.
6 months	Brings hand to mouth.
8 to 9 months	Holds and plays with spoon
9 months	Holds bottle or breast, drinks from glass held for him.
10 months	Finger-feeds self.
11 to 14 months	Chews and swallows solid foods; appetite decreases.
12 to 16 months	Holds cup with two hands and drinks.
15 months	Begins to feed self with spoon held in fist.
18 months	Feeds self with spoon held in fist without spilling much (may still prefer finger-feeding).
22 months	Unwraps food.
24 months	Decreased need for animal fats.
28 months	Feeds self with fork held in fist (may still prefer finger-feeding).
30 months	Drinks from straw with assistance.
36 months	Eats with fork and spoon held underhand, sits in chair throughout meal.
42 months	Drinks from cup or glass held with one hand, uses napkin, cleans up own spills.
45 months	Serves self from serving bowl.
48 months	Clears setting from table after meal, chews with mouth closed, spreads food with knife.
54 months	Cuts food with fork, passes serving bowl.
60 months	Helps set table.

TOILET TRAINING

A toilet-trained child is considerably easier to care for than a child who is still dependent upon diapers. Therefore, parents are understandably interested in having their child achieve bowel and bladder control as soon as possible. But it is also true that our society is obsessed with being first and best. This obsession seems to carry over into the realm of toilet training: parents tend to want their child to be the first to be toilet-trained among their circle of friends.

How will parents know when their child's nervous system is developed well enough so toilet training can begin? When a child is able to stand up without assistance, his spinal cord is fairly well developed and he will begin to make certain physical movements, words, or sounds in anticipation of defecating or urinating. This usually occurs around the end of the first year and marks the earliest age at which toilet training should be considered. It is crucial, however, that the child be old enough to understand what the parents are asking him to do, which may necessitate waiting until after one year of age.

Toilet training usually follows this sequence: 1) bowel control at night, 2) bowel control during the day, 3) bladder control during the day, 4) bladder control at night. Bowel control training, therefore, should be undertaken first and bladder training should be withheld until about one month later.

How does a parent go about toilet training a child? The first step is to determine the child's schedule of bowel movements. For a few weeks, a record can be kept of when bowel movement occurs. If the child is free from illness, and if abrupt changes in diet or eating schedule do not occur, a pattern should appear so that parents can predict approximately what time of day the child will have a movement. Once such a regular pattern emerges, training can begin.

Shortly before the time a child is expected to have a bowel movement, he can be seated on the potty (a child-sized potty, of which he is not afraid) in a room free from distractions. The child is told what is expected of him in a casual, matter-of-fact way, consistently using one word which he will understand to mean having a bowel movement. When the child defecates, he should be praised profusely for his act, making it clear exactly what the praise is for. By praising the act ("you did a good job") instead of the child ("you were a good boy"), the child will not feel that he is a good person only when he has a bowel movement (there are plenty of other occasions during the day for praising the child). When he does not have a movement disappointment or disapproval should not be evident, there will be a next time. After bowel control is accomplished, bladder training proceeds in the same way. After determining the child's natural schedule, he is taken to the potty when he is expected to urinate, praised when he succeeds, and not scolded for failures.

The entire process of toilet training often takes as long as two years. The average child will achieve bowel control by about 18 months, daytime bladder control by two years of age, and nighttime bladder control by age three. Developmental norms must be remembered. Because a child is a little late he is not abnormal. Regarding daytime bladder control, there need not be concern unless the child is not fairly well trained by age four. Table 6-2 shows the percentages of children of various ages who still have occasional accidents or occasionally wet the bed.

Table 6-2
Percentage of Children Not Totally Bladder-Trained at Various Ages

Age	Percent Not Trained
2	90
4–5	20
6–7	13
14	2

7 Social-Emotional Development

Perhaps no aspect of a child's development is as gratifying to parents as his becoming a feeling, interacting, social human being. The purpose of this section is to describe the warp in which the simple world of the infant turns into the rich, complex, social and emotional world of the adult.

THE EMERGENCE OF SELF

A child comes into the world with no sense that he is a creature separate and apart from other objects and creatures. One of his first tasks is to learn the difference between "me" and "not me." He becomes aware of the movements of his own body. He begins to recognize internal changes such as hunger. He learns that when he makes sounds, he not only feels sensations in his throat, but also hears the sounds at the same time. He observes how his behavior affects objects around him. As a result of activities such as these, he develops an awareness of his physical self and its separations from that which is not part of himself.

Infants seem to come into the world capable of experiencing only one emotion: generalized excitement. There are wide individual differences in both the activity level and the emotional responsiveness of infants. Some children are naturally more active than others. Some react to stimulation with more excitement and agitation than others do. These individual differences seem to be "built-in."

Gradually the child's repertoire of emotions increases and his emotional reactions become increasingly differentiated. Some time around the age of three months other emotions can be identified.

ATTACHMENT-SEPARATION

Crying and social smiling signal the addition to the infant's emotional repertoire of distress and delight. These behaviors are also a part of another process, bonding, or attachment to mother or to a mother substitute. At first, attachment behaviors occur more or less automatically, and in response to any human being. Because the young infant cannot differentiate between different people he can change mothers (as in the case of adoption) with no harmful effects. Around the age of two or three months, however, the child begins to learn to tell different people apart, and his attachment behaviors then begin to occur primarily in response to one person, or at the most, a few people. He is still friendly to strangers, but he prefers the company of only a few special people. Another change occurs around the age of six months. The child's ability to get around by himself is improving by this age, and his mental development is approaching the stage when he can form mental images of people: out of sight no longer means out of mind. Thus, he will start to take the initiative in gaining and maintaining proximity and contact. His attachment behaviors are no longer automatic and disjointed; they become intentional and well integrated.

The attachment process is an extremely important aspect of human development. In fact, child psychologist John Bowlby has stated that the major task of the first three years of life is to form an attachment to at least one other human being. This is necessary if an infant is to survive in the world, as well as for another important reason. The bond between mother and child serves as the prototype for the child's affectional relationships throughout the rest of his life. In essence, people learn how to love during the first years of their lives in the context of this bond. A healthy bond between the two is a necessary foundation for healthy love relationships later on.

A healthy attachment relationship is a two-way relationship. Mother and child need each other, love each other, and each derives pleasure from interacting with the other. This is in contrast to dependency, which is a one-sided relationship in which a child depends on mother for fulfillment of his needs, and his behavior is controlled by mother. Dependency is one-sided; attachment is mutually satisfying. The relationship between the very young infant and its mother resembles a dependency relationship, but as the child matures and the bonding process follows its course, dependency decreases and a reciprocal attachment develops.

As the child's attachment to mother increases, his reactions to strangers turn from indiscriminately positive to neutral and finally to strongly negative. By progressing through a series of stages, the child develops a fear of strangers which is often confused with "separation anxiety." Although these two phenomena emerge at about the same time, they are quite different things. Fear of strangers refers to a negative reaction to the presence of unfamiliar people. Separation anxiety is an uncomfortable feeling resulting from being physically separated from mother, regardless of whether or not strangers are present. Separation anxiety is usually present between the ages of seven months and two or three years, during which time the child is torn between two opposing tendencies. On the one hand, he feels a need to explore his environment. His ability to get around by himself allows him to do this, and this is how he develops intellectually. On the other hand, he feels a strong attachment to mother and does not want to leave her. His solution to this dilemma is to use mother as a secure base from which to explore. As long as mother stays in one place and keeps her attention on her child, the child will move about and explore the area. However, as soon as mother gets up and moves, or turns her attention to someone else, the child will quickly return to her. Outdoors, most children will wander about 200 feet from mother to explore, but will return to her periodically.

Most of what we have said about the development of an attachment between mother and child is summarized in Table 7-1. This table shows how behaviors toward mothers and behaviors toward strangers complement each other at each age level.

Table 7-1
The Chronological Development of Attachment
Between Mother and Child

Age	Child's Attachment Behavior	
	Toward Mother	Toward Strangers
0 to 1 month	Reflex smiling.	Reflect smiling.
1 to 2 months	"Social smile": gives full smile while looking person in the eye.	Cannot discriminate between people; responds to anyone with "social smile": no fear of strangers.
3 to 5 months	"Selective social smile": smile and other attachment behaviors directed primarily to one or a few special people.	Can discriminate between familiar people and strangers, but no fear of strangers; approaches strangers haphazardly.
5 to 6 months	Develops internal representation of mother: takes active initiative in seeking proximity to mother.	Sobers and stares at sight of stranger, but no real fear.
7 months	Uses mother as secure base from which to explore; shows "separation anxiety": follows mother when she leaves; cries if he cannot follow her; greets mother when she returns.	Uneasy around strangers.

Table 7-1 *(continued)*

8 months		Active fear of strangers: restlessness, loud crying, withdrawal.
9 to 10 months		Fear of strangers reaches peak intensity.
12 to 15 months		Offers and releases objects to stranger.
15 to 18 months	Accepts brief absence.	Will play briefly with stranger.
18 to 21 months	Accepts explained absence.	Has "favorite" adults.
21 to 24 months	Accepts absence.	Is curious about strangers.
2 to 3 years	Develops insight into mother's feelings and behavior; separation anxiety disappears.	

THE DEVELOPMENT OF SELF-CONCEPT, SELF-ESTEEM

We previously mentioned that children are born with no real sense of being unique creatures who are separate from their environments. By experiencing the effects of environmental stimulation on various parts of their bodies and by observing the effects of various parts of their bodies on objects around them, infants gradually learn to distinguish "me" from "not me." The 12-week-old baby will regard his own hand as part of himself. The 24-week-old infant will smile and vocalize at his image in a mirror. The 30-month-old child will refer to himself with the pronoun "I." Thus the child is developing a sense of being a separate and unique person.

A child's physical characteristics and motor skills are important early determinants of self-concept and self-esteem. If he perceives his physical appearance and abilities positively and if he experiences success in motor tasks, his self-esteem will be enhanced. If a child has a physical deformity, his self-concept will be affected; he will be aware that he is physically different from others. However, whether or not his overall self-esteem will be affected depends on the kind of feedback he receives from others. He may come to believe that "Because I have a defective body, I am a defective person," or he may learn "Even though I look different and I can't do certain things, I'm still a valuable, worthwhile, lovable person."

Another aspect of the young child's developing self-concept relates to his growing independence. Between the time when the mother-child attachment bond reaches its peak and the time when the child begins school the child's relationships with his mother and with his environment change. His attachment with mother decreases and is replaced with a more mature partnership relationship. This relationship is more cooperative, more balanced, more "give and take" than the previous attachment. The child becomes less egocentric: he realizes that mother has goals and needs also and is able to see the world from her point of view.

Concurrent with the decrease in attachment and development of a partnership relationship is an increase in independence. Around age four to four and one-half years, there is a sudden decline in separation anxiety, and the child no longer needs mother as a secure base from which to explore. He will begin to explore and master his environment independently and learn to take care of himself in the world.

The success which the child attains achieving this new autonomy will affect his self-concept. As he independently encounters the new aspects of his environment, he must make decisions and test his skills. If he is encouraged to try new things, praised for his success, and reassured after failures, he is likely to think of himself as a competent, autonomous child. If, on the other hand, his independence is discouraged and his efforts are belittled, he will begin to doubt his own competence, and he will remain dependent and in need of support from others.

During the preschool period, when the child is reducing his dependence on mother and increasing his independence endeavors, he typically begins to enter social situations. Social interactions with peers provide the child with a chance to try out what he has learned from his family in a new situation. From his interactions with his parents, the child has a preliminary sense of what kind of person he is. From the particular structure of his family (that is, the number and ages of brothers and sisters), the child has had practice interacting with certain kinds of people. When the child begins interacting with peers, he tries to apply his fledging social skills and self-concept in this new setting. Peers then provide a new "social mirror," from which the child receives additional feedback regarding the kind of person he is. So, while the family's influences on the child affect how he interacts with his peers, the peers also influence the child, and this influence filters back into the family.

SOCIALIZATION

The child's early experiences in learning social skills occur in the family. While interacting with his parents, brothers, and sisters, the child is indoctrinated with "dos" and "don'ts." He sees his parents and siblings interact with each other, and he imitates what he sees. He is rewarded for certain acts and punished for others. His family determines what kinds of experiences, books, television programs, people, and toys he is exposed to. Through these types of experiences the child begins to learn some social skills. He learns how to take care of himself so that others will accept him. He learns the language skills necessary to communicate with other people. He learns how to approach people of different ages and genders, how to get along with people of different temperaments, and how to deal with the same people in different situations. He learns what forms of emotional expression are acceptable. For example, temper tantrums may be acceptable in one family and taboo in another, verbal expressions of anger may be acceptable where physical tantrums are not, or emotional expressions may be outlawed in any form. The child also learns attitudes toward a wide variety of topics, such as foods, music, race, and religion. These attitudes will affect who a child associates with and how he interacts with people.

If this early learning is adequate, the child is likely to get along well with peers later on. If, on the other hand, the child does not have adequate opportunities to interact with his family and learn social skills, the result is likely to be a downward cycle. The child will be ill equipped to get along with peers and will tend to avoid contact with them. He then misses out on more opportunities to learn social skills, and his deficit becomes even greater.

As they get older, there is a general trend for children to interact more and more with peers and less and less with adults. Thus, as children mature more and more of the burden of learning social skills is spent on those in their age group. Children learn to get along with each other through the medium of play. Before the age of two children do not interact with each other but play independently by themselves. Even if two young children are placed together, they will play independently, as if they were alone. Around age three children begin to engage in "parallel play." At this stage they play near each other, are aware of each other's presence and actions, and will imitate each other. For example, two boys may play "army," watching each other and imitating each other's actions. But each will be playing army more or less independently: they will not interact with each other as "good guy" and "bad guy." Throughout the preschool parallel play years children learn to share playthings with each other. They gradually begin to assign differentiated roles to each other: for example, "cops and robbers" or "cowboys and Indians." They begin to be selective in choosing friends.

When infants are born they are neither moral nor immoral; they are not concerned about the positive or negative consequences of their actions on others. When they begin to progress beyond the infant stage, children begin to adjust their behavior according to the demands of other people. For example, the toddler learns that he can no longer defecate when and where he wants to; he must defecate when and where his parents want him to. By watching and listening to adults the young child begins to acquire information about the ways in which he is expected to behave. He finds that he is praised and rewarded for behaving as his parents want him to, while he is punished, scolded, or ignored when he misbehaves or fails to behave as expected. As he grows older, peers and teachers join his parents in this teaching process. This is often called the age of *external controls:* the child's behavior is controlled by other people. He behaves in a certain way in a certain situation because he believes that that behavior will earn him the greatest reward. His "moral" behavior represents the action of forces outside of himself; he has no internal behavior controls or moral principles.

Over a period of time, however, the child begins to "internalize" codes which have been imposed upon him. That is, he develops some sort of internal sense of how he is supposed to behave. An example will serve to illustrate the difference between this stage, the stage of *internal controls,* and the previous one. The younger child may learn that if he gets into the cookie jar while Mom is in the kitchen his hand will be slapped. He wisely avoids the cookie jar when Mom is around. However, when she is upstairs, the child may raid the cookie jar with no real sense that he is doing anything wrong. The older child, on the other hand, if he has "internalized" the rule about staying out of the cookie jar, will follow the rule even when Mom is absent and he has little chance of getting caught. He learns to resist temptation, or if he fails to resist the temptation, he will know that he is breaking a rule, and he will probably feel guilty.

A child learns to control his behavior first, during the stage of external controls. Then, during the stage of internal controls, an emotional component enters the picture. The child feels anxious when he thinks about misbehaving and guilty after he misbehaves. There is a third aspect of the development of social controls: making intellectual judgments about behavior. Here, we are talking about morals and "morality." We may say that a person is "morally mature" when he is able to make decisions and judgments based on internal principles and when he acts in accordance with these judgments. Morality develops slowly and does not become mature until early adolescence. Although children know society's basic rules by the first grade, their ability to make moral judgments develops slowly and in stages. The development of personal controls and morality is summarized in Table 7-2.

ENHANCING SOCIAL-EMOTIONAL DEVELOPMENT

The following suggestions are made directly to mothers, for enhancing the child's social-emotional development. They relate especially to aspects of social-emotional development that have been discussed.

- Pick up your young infant and cradle him often. Do not be afraid to "ham it up" with plenty of crooning. Enjoy your infant and let him enjoy you. Physical contact between infant and caretaker is important for both physical and emotional development. The lack of adequate contact in infancy can lead to an emotionally impoverished life.

Table 7-2
Stages in Development of Personal Controls and Morality

Stage	Age Span	Characteristics of Stage
Amorality	Infant	Acts for own well-being; disregards effects on others; no awareness of morality.
External controls	Toddler and preschool	Adjusts behavior to the demands of others in order to get rewards and avoid punishment; sense of morality is geared to result of behavior.
Internal controls	Preschool and early school years	Fears punishment and feels guilty after misbehaving; resists temptations, controls or inhibits behavior, sense of morality no longer dependent on immediate consequences.
Premoral, moral realism	Prominent before age 10; then decreases with age	Accepts superior power, rules seen as universal and absolute; how "bad" an act is depends on its consequences.
A) Punishment and obedience orientation		Obeys rules to avoid punishment.
B) Naive instrumental morality		Obeys rules to obtain rewards.

Morality of emotional role. Conformity, moral subjectivism.	Increases until age 13, then stabilizes and remains predominant	Rules are flexible conventions that help people get along with each other; how bad an act is depends on intent.
A) Good-boy morality		Conforms to obtain the approval and avoid the disapproval of others.
B) Authority-maintaining morality		Sense of duty to authority; conforms to avoid official censure and subsequent guilt.
Morality of self-accepted moral principles	Increases between ages 13 and 16 in some individuals; remains secondary to previous stage; may never develop.	
A) Morality or contract		Focuses on individual rights, democratically accepted law, and community welfare; sense of obligation to group; conforms to maintain community respect.
B) Morality of individual principles or conscience		Follows internal principles; conforms to these principles to avoid self-condemnation.

- Provide your infant with plenty of safe, attractive toys and objects to manipulate. He learns the difference between "me" and "not me" by manipulating his environment. Give him the opportunity to do this.
- A young child's emotional world is relatively simple, and he demands a lot from you without being able to give much back. This is normal. Try not to expect more of your child than he is able to give. If it often seems that your child's demands are just too much for you, it may be that you have an unusually demanding child, but it may also be that you need to find new ways of meeting his needs.
- Foster a strong mother-child attachment. A strong emotional bond between mother and child during the first year of life is important; this is where the child learns to love, to be loved, and to trust people. At this age, do not be afraid to respond to your child's need, this will not "spoil" him!
- From about seven months to two or three years of age, your child will explore his environment, while using mother as a secure base from which to explore. Encourage him to do this. Allow him to wander as much as safety and convenience will allow, but let him know that you are still there when he needs you. This will allow him to develop a sense of independence and competence.
- During your child's preschool years continue to encourage him to explore and try out new things. He will have less need for you as a base of operations by this stage. Encourage him to begin playing with other children. Praise him when he succeeds at something; reassure him when he fails. In this way he will learn the preliminary social skills that will start him on his way toward feeling adequate, competent, and worthwhile.
- For a child to develop a healthy self-concept, he must believe that he is worthwhile, lovable, and generally OK. The way you discipline your child is crucial in enhancing a positive self-concept. He must be disciplined in order to learn to control his behavior and get along socially, but he must also receive consistent "I love you" and "you are OK" messages. The ideal situation is one where the parent delivers consistent "you are worthwhile" messages and adequate discipline. The rules and limits which you set for your child should be clear to everyone involved. You should specify what the child is or is not to do, why you think it is important that he behave that way, what the consequences will be if he fails to conform to the rule, and how (and by whom) these consequences will be administered. The rules should be negotiable: everyone in

your family should have input into setting and modifying the rules. By clearly stating the rules and making them negotiable you guard against the danger that they will outlive their usefulness.

PART II

Handicapped Growth

8 Handicapping Conditions

In the first part of this book the development of the normal child was considered, focusing on physical, mental, motor, and neurologic growth.

Two of the handicapping conditions that may afflict children will now be discussed: developmental disabilities and developmental delay. Succeeding chapters will deal with specific handicapping conditions such as mental retardation, cerebral palsy, epilepsy, emotional and psychological problems, and learning disabilities. We will attempt to direct inquiries to suggested readings and professional agencies where greater depth of information may be obtained.

The term developmental disability is used to designate a broad range of handicaps occurring in children. These are chronic and impose some functional limitation on the child. A child with a developmental disability may have one single handicapping condition, for example, deafness, or he may have multiple handicaps, perhaps cerebral palsy with hearing loss and mental retardation. These conditions may be congenital or hereditary (genetic). They may be caused by accident, infection, birth trauma, or numerous other insults.

SOME DEFINITIONS

For better comprehension, it is necessary to define some of the terms. (See also the Glossary at the end of the book.) *Congenital* means being present at birth. *Hereditary* refers to the transmission of a given trait from parents to their children. A cleft lip and palate can be inherited and are congenital, because they are both present at birth and usually inherited. A *torsion* or twisting of the lower leg in a newborn infant is congenital because it is present at birth but is not inherited. *Huntington's chorea,* on the other hand, is not congenital as it is not manifest at birth, but is an inherited disease that manifests itself in midlife.

The definition of developmental disabilities has been extended to include not only the mentally retarded and children with cerebral palsy, but also people with epilepsy, learning disabilities, congenital malformations, and many other difficulties occurring during the developmental period of childhood. In November 1978 President Carter signed into law bill number 95-602, which established a new legal definition of developmental disabilities. This bill, using a functional definition calls a developmental disability:

> Severe, chronic disability which is attributable to a mental or physical impairment or combination of mental and physical impairments ...manifested before age 22; which is likely to continue indefinitely, which results in substantial functional limitations in certain specific areas and which reflects the need for lifelong individually planned services.

The House of Representatives revised the definition in the existing law by specifying the disabilities that would constitute a developmental disability. This law was extended beyond the previously-covered children with mental retardation, cerebral palsy, epilepsy, learning disabilities, and congenital malformations to cover all children with severe, chronic disability.

Handicapping conditions that may occur in children are many and varied. They may be small or extensive. They may involve one organ system such as the brain or heart, several organ systems such as the brain and liver, or they may affect the entire body. Generally, disabilities involving more than one organ system tend to be more complex and tend to create greater functional difficulties for the child.

Specific subjects such as mental retardation, cerebral palsy, epilepsy, emotional and psychological problems, learning disabilities, and congenital abnormalities will be discussed in this section. It is imperative to make clear to the reader that guidelines for handicapping conditions must be broad. What is a handicap to one child may be no handicap, or at most a minor nuisance to another child, depending on the severity of the involvement.

The concerned parent needs to be reminded that if a child has a condition which seems outside the range of broad guidelines for normalcy, professional help must be secured before a definitive diagnosis can be obtained. Only after the diagnosis is made can a treatment program be outlined medically, socially, psychologically, and educationally to help the child develop to his greatest potential.

The history of social concerns for the handicapped child has been extremely interesting. In some primitive societies any child born with a handicap, particularly an obvious physical handicap, eg, a missing arm or leg, cleft lip or palate, or an obvious facial abnormality, was immediately destroyed. In other societies he was deified and worshipped. Even in more sophisticated societies the attitude toward the handicapped has been kind in some eras and cruel in others. At times, they have been eagerly sought as talismans or good luck charms for the nobility; at other times they have been cast into dungeons with the criminally insane or castigated and scourged as products of Satan.

It has only been in the past one hundred years that the world has made any attempt to diagnose the cause of disabilities and to institute wherever possible, treatment and educational programs to bring these once-scorned children out of the closets and permit them to participate in life's activities with their peers to the full extent of their capabilities.

SURVEY OF DEVELOPMENTAL DISABILITIES

Let us look briefly at the general concept of developmental disabilities—what are they, how they are diagnosed, the means of treatment, and methods of prevention available to us today.

Congenital malformations are structural malformations of the body present at birth. These may be gross or microscopic, external so they can be seen, or within the body itself. They may be single, they may be multiple; they may be hereditary or nonhereditary.

Today, approximately 5% of infants born in the United States are born with some type of congenital defect. This rate probably has not appreciably changed since records were first accumulated at the turn of the century.

The study of these congenital malformations has led to the development of a new specialty. Dysmorphology is a term that has recently been introduced to identify the general category of diseases that accompany congenital abnormalities (in structural tissues) regardless of the cause or severity. Teratogen or teratogenic are also useful terms when referring to something having the capability of producing malformations in the child during prenatal development.

To date a number of environmental influences that can have an adverse effect on the developing embryo have been identified. Table 8-1 lists a few of the environmental teratogens capable of causing embryonic damage if taken by mothers at a certain time of pregnancy and if the child is genetically susceptible. There is no way of determining which children are susceptible to these insults. It must be emphasized that any given one of these environmental drugs or diseases may not cause difficulties in all pregnancies. The most severe damage usually occurs if the insult occurs during the first trimester, approximately the first 12 to 14 weeks of pregnancy.

Some of the teratogens appear to have no effect after the first trimester, eg, thalidomide and rubella, while others can have a damaging effect because of their continual or recurrent insult to the fetus through the entire pregnancy, eg, diabetes mellitus and alcohol. These effects are discussed later in the chapter.

62

Table 8-1
Environmental Teratogens

Medication Taken by the Mother
  Thalidomide
  Aminopterin
  Amethopterin
  Hormones—some progestins, androgens, and even estrogens

Medications Considered Suspect
  Phenytoin (Dilantin)
  Lithium
  Quinine
  Hydrocortisone or other steroids
  Coumarin and its derivatives
  Trimethadione
  Amphetamine
  LSD and other hallucinogenics

Maternal Metabolic Disease
  Diabetes mellitus
  Phenylpyruvic oligophrenia

Alcohol

Ionizing Irradiation
  Therapeutic pelvic x-rays
  Exposure to severe high-dosage irradiation

Viruses
  Rubella (German measles)
  Toxoplasmosis
  Cytomegalovirus
  Questionably significant: mumps, rubeola (red measles), infectious hepatitis, influenza
  Other viral agents such as herpes simplex, infectious mononucleosis, poliomyelitis, vaccinia (smallpox), and varicella (chicken pox) may cause serious fetal disease but do not necessarily lead to congenital malformations.

Other Infections
  Syphilis

    The list in Table 8-1 is by no means complete, and many determinations are being made today of new possible teratogenic agents.
    The precise etiology of a single malformation is seldom clear, since the fundamental cause appears to differ in individuals evidencing the same type of malformation. Genetic causes appear to play a major role, and it is felt that congenital malformations are approximately 20% inherited, 20% due to environmental factors, and 60% due to combined genetic and environmental factors.

In cases of children with multiple malformations a distinctive pattern sometimes emerges, which constitutes a specific entity. This is then called a syndrome. Many of these syndromes of abnormalities appear to be genetically determined.

Another significant condition a dysmorphologist will look for is the presence of minor congenital malformations consisting of structural changes which have little or no medical consequence and are frequently overlooked and relatively insignificant. These might include minor changes of the position of the ears, changes in the hands, widening of the eyes, and webbing between the fingers and toes. The correlation of many of these minor findings with other major defects helps establish the diagnosis of many of the malformation syndromes.

DIAGNOSTIC PROCEDURES

What are the diagnostic procedures involved in determining the presence or absence of potential developmental disabilities in a child?

A systematic evaluation of the history, physical findings and, where indicated, laboratory data, are utilized to arrive at this type of diagnosis. A comprehensive history of the child and his prenatal history is, perhaps, the beginning point of an evaluation. A thorough search should be made through the mother's history as to the presence or absence of any environmental insults—medications, drugs, illnesses, bleeding, difficulty of any kind occurring with her pregnancy. Were there difficulties at the time of birth? Were the baby's heart tones monitored, and if so, were there significant changes in the baby's heart rate during labor? Did the baby respond well immediately after birth? Did he cry and breathe spontaneously, did the muscle tone return as anticipated? What has been the developmental history to date? Has the child's muscle tone always been good? Did he hold his head up, sit, walk, and talk in accordance with the guidelines discussed in the previous section of this book? What types of symptoms is the child having at the present time? What are the parents' concerns, worries, and fears? These should all be imparted to the health professional.

In most cases, a complete pedigree of the family history should be taken in order to identify other individuals in the family having any dysmorphology, mental retardation, or other known disabilities.

The child should be examined thoroughly with a complete physical and neurological examination. Where indicated, special laboratory tests should be ordered.

An EEG, or brain wave tracing, might be done to determine whether there is a normal pattern. X-rays might be taken of the head, arms, legs, hips, or any other abnormal areas. In certain cases, computerized axial tomography, radiosound, or other sophisticated diagnostic procedures might be indicated.

At the present time, the majority of states in the United States are doing neonatal screening, and laws have been presented to Congress to make this mandatory in all 50 states. Present screening in most states is limited to screening for phenylketonuria (PKU). In some states hypothyroidism, which has an occurrence rate twice that of PKU, galactosemia, maple syrup urine disease, and other of the aminoacidurias, which are discussed later in this book, are part of the newborn screening.

Such screening is not done in all states at the present time, and it should be encouraged, as these diseases are usually treatable if found within the first two to three weeks of life. Severe brain damage will occur if diagnosis and institution of treatment are delayed.

Many studies are available to show that these screening tests are cost-effective. A recent report from the Comptroller General of the United States has shown that the cost of caring for these defective children, if untreated, far exceeds the cost of screening all children born in the United States.

The influence of our modern environment with its smog and other air pollutions has not been fully evaluated at this time. A compilation of statistics since the turn of the century has shown a relatively continuous 5% incidence of congenital malformations. Because of the relatively static incidence, most people feel that these environmental influences play a minor role, if any, in the production of congenital malformations. Careful studies have not been done in this area, and good data need to be collected.

PREVENTION

What are our present available options for the prevention of developmental disabilities?

Several options have been instituted and are effecting a reduction in the incidence of many disabilities. Good prenatal care has been effective in reducing the incidence of prematurity and birth trauma. Kernicterus, once frequent with Rh incompatibility, is almost a thing of the past.

Comprehensive newborn care with good general newborn nurseries has had good effect. Where needed, intensive care nurseries for the care of the children in severe distress, and the comprehensive care of prematures have resulted in reduced mortality and disabilities.

More and more effort is being put into identifying and reducing environmental poisonings, particularly those occurring from lead intoxication. Children are extremely susceptible to this type of intoxication and can sustain severe brain damage. Paints used in older homes in years past all contained lead as their principal source of pigment. Children were frequently known to eat peeling paint, and the incidence of lead poisoning was frequent. Paints used inside houses today no longer contain lead which has resulted in a marked reduction in the incidence of this type of lead intoxication. In certain mining communities, pollution from mineral extraction processes resulted in the contamination of water supplies by lead compounds, with resulting high incidences of lead poisoning. Better control of the extraction wastes and the prevention of contamination of culinary water sources has reduced the incidence of lead poisoning in children in these areas. There is still much to be done, and environmental controls still remain necessary.

The increasing availability of genetic counseling, either through family physicians, pediatricians, or genetic centers, has made it possible for people with known genetic disease to receive proper counseling prior to making decisions as to the size of their families.

Termination of a pregnancy shown to be producing a defective child adds to our prevention. Though the subject of therapeutic abortion remains an ethical issue, it is a sound medical alternative.

IMMUNIZATION

Immunizations for prevention of disease are extremely important in preventing serious consequences of diseases capable of infecting the embryo or fetus during pregnancy. Infections caused by many of these preventable diseases can cause severe damage, malformations, or even fetal death. The latest immunization survey by the Center for Disease Control (CDC) confirms that barely two-thirds of children aged one to four years throughout the United States have full protection from all diseases avoidable by vaccination. The levels of adult protection are even lower. The avoidable diseases are tetanus, diphtheria, pertussis (whooping cough), poliomyelitis, measles, rubella (German measles), and mumps. It is true that there are certain risks to immunization, but these are extremely slight. Risks perhaps increase when live-virus vaccine preparations are used. It is important, however, to separate true allergic reactions to vaccine, which are rare, from minor reactions or from unrelated problems such as symptoms of a concurrent disease or illness.

There are valid reasons for postponing and, in some cases, not giving immunizations, but such cases are extremely rare. Individual determinations must be made by a physician. An acute febrile illness warrants postponement. When there is a minor respiratory illness, it might be wise to wait a day or two to be sure that the illness does not become serious before giving the immunization.

A child likely to have an allergic reaction to a vaccine should not receive it, but the parent and doctor should be certain of the child's allergic history before the vaccine is withheld. For example, no adverse effects should be anticipated in an egg-sensitive child from giving live measles virus vaccine, since the virus is not grown in eggs but is grown in fibroblast tissue cultures so that the egg albumen and yolk are not present.

Vaccines containing live viruses are definitely contraindicated in children with immunodeficiency diseases (children whose immune mechanism is abnormal). Also, routine immunization of children taking any medications that suppress the immune mechanism, or the cortisone drugs or drugs used to treat leukemias and other cancer problems should be deferred until therapy is completed. There is, however, no need to withhold therapy with the inactivated vaccines such as DPT (diphtheria, pertussis, and tetanus). Even though the incidence of these diseases in the United States has decreased markedly in the past 20 years, they are still prevalent and capable of causing difficulty.

For the nine-month period through October 7, 1978, there were still 62 cases of diphtheria, 24,000 cases of measles (rubeola), 1600 cases of pertussis (whooping cough), almost 17,000 cases of rubella (German measles), 64 cases of tetanus, and two cases of poliomyelitis reported in the United States. In addition to this, 17,000 cases of syphilis have been reported—a disease which can cause severe congenital malformations and brain damage. During this same period 23 cases of congenital rubella were reported in the United States in spite of the availability of good rubella vaccines. These diseases are probably underreported and do not represent the total number of actual cases occurring within the United States.

In rubella the primary concern is preventing the development of congenital rubella in the unborn child. This can be accomplished by ensuring that all women in the child-bearing age either have received their immunizations or are properly immunized prior to the onset of pregnancy.

National morbidity data show that both rubella infection and congenital rubella have declined in frequency. An epidemic occurring in 1964 and 1965 produced more than 20,000 newborns with congenital rubella, a significant portion of whom had severe congenital malformations.

In spite of some controversy as to the best time for immunization for rubella, there is still good reason to feel that young children, preferably beyond 15 months of age, should receive a primary immunization. We also should be sure that target groups not initially protected, such as young girls approaching the child-bearing age, should be immunized. Laboratory tests presently available can determine the amount of protection an individual has by examining the blood serum for the presence of antibodies to rubella. If these are in inadequate supply, immunization in most cases should be recommended several months prior to conception. Present recommendations advise against active immunization during pregnancy, as there is some concern about the transfer of the attenuated live virus to the fetus. In the United States no cases of congenital rubella have been reported to date that were caused by an immunization given during the early weeks of pregnancy. (In many cases the woman was not aware that she was pregnant.) The recommendations, however, are that a woman should probably wait for at least three months after active immunization before attempting to conceive.

It is extremely important that children with developmental disabilities receive their routine immunizations unless there is some marked contraindication. In the process of seeing, evaluating, and caring for a disabled child, many times the routine immunizations are neglected or overlooked. These children are equally, or even more susceptible, to these common infections.

Special questions regarding revaccinations, special immunizations required for travel in certain parts of the world, and contraindications should be discussed with a health professional.

Table 8-2 is a suggested schedule for children's immunizations.

Table 8-2
Schedule of Primary and Secondary Immunizations

Age	Vaccines	Comments
	Primary Immunizations	
2 months	DPT and polio	DPT—Diphtheria, pertussis (whooping cough), and tetanus
4 months	DPT and polio	Polio—trivalent oral polio vaccine (TOPV)
6 months	DPT	Polio dose is optional
15 months	Measles, mumps, rubella	Usually combined as the M-R or M-M-R shot; may be given separately.
18 months	DPT and polio	These doses are considered an integral part of the primary immunization series.
	Booster Immunizations	
4 to 6 years	DPT and polio	Preferably given prior to day care or school entry.
Every 10 years	TD (adult)	Tetanus-diphtheria for persons age six years and older should be given at ten-year intervals.

THERAPY OF DEVELOPMENTAL DISABILITIES

A time-honored procedure in treating the developmentally disabled consists of the surgical repair of congenital malformations wherever possible. Cleft lips and palates are now being repaired at an early age at least with primary closure, and long-term results in the hands of good plastic surgeons have been excellent.

The surgical repair of congenital malformations of the heart has progressed rapidly during the past two decades. Open heart surgery on infants, once deemed impossible, is now performed routinely in indicated cases. Surgical morbidity and mortality have decreased as techniques have been improved and more surgeons have been trained. The addition of the open-heart bypass equipment permitting careful surgery on an open heart has extended the possibilities of cure to many severe defects.

Surgical procedures are used, of course, to remove skin abnormalities where possible. Extra fingers, toes, reconstruction of ears, noses, and for that matter entire faces are now being reconstructed where needed. For many malformations, artificial joints and improved orthopedic surgical techniques have all added to decrease the child's long-term physical limitations.

Parallel to this has come the development of better prostheses, artificial arms and legs. The arrival of the true "bionic man" is not here, but the prosthetic equipment being developed throughout the world is progressing rapidly.

Coupled with the development of these prosthetic devices is a group of professionals who work with the children to teach them to use their artificial limbs properly. They are trained to fit the limbs and teach the children to use them, and they follow the patients throughout childhood modifying and changing the artificial arms and legs as becomes necessary.

The medical approaches to treatment of disabilities again have progressed rapidly. Today we are able to treat many of the rare inborn errors of metabolism with diet modification. Treatment with these modified diets has proved to be extremely efficient in preventing the severe mental retardation which can occur with these diseases.

Better treatment for children with diabetes, more careful monitoring and control, better medications, and perhaps the promise in the future of the development of human insulin from recombinant DNA experimentation is within the grasp of medical science.

Children today are protected from acute infectious illnesses either by immunizations, vaccinations, or by active treatment with antibiotics. Rheumatic fever, a frequent disease four decades ago, has been reduced markedly by the use of antibiotics in treating "strep" throats. It is almost a rarity today, and the complication of acute rheumatic heart disease is a rarity in clinical practice.

Virus diseases not responsive to antibiotics can be prevented with certain vaccines as in the case of poliomyelitis. Good symptomatic treatment of the infection will prevent serious disability from occurring in many cases.

The medical management of sickle cell disease, thalassemia, and other blood abnormalities, though not totally effective to date, has improved and the morbidity associated with these diseases has lessened.

Intervention with special education is the most effective therapeutic program in treating the mentally retarded child. Unfortunately, for the vast majority of cases of mental retardation there is no known effective medical program available today. Exceptions are those few cases of mental retardation due to PKU or some other inborn error of metabolism or due to cretinism. Diet therapy often corrects the former, and cretinism is responsive to thyroid hormone replacement.

To repeat—for most mentally retarded children special education is the ultimate mode of therapy. It is imperative that these children be developed to the full extent of their capabilities. Special educators assisted by specialists in the areas of speech, hearing, physical, and occupational therapy have the capabilities of developing their potential. Early intervention programs, both for preschool and school-age children, and special educational techniques have been designed and developed to help the handicapped child, whether retarded or normal, and all are being employed to offer better life for the child in the future.

Psychologic intervention is important in counseling the child and perhaps more important, in counseling members of his family to help them comprehend and understand the child's disability. The family members must understand the disease, its genetic implications if there are any, their feelings, anxieties, angers, and guilt feelings that are expressed toward the disabled child. In most situations, counseling need not be extensive and can be handled fairly easily by most health professionals. In cases of severe emotional responses to the disabled child, comprehensive counseling with a psychologist or psychiatrist might be necessary.

Treatment of the developmentally disabled has progressed rapidly in the past two decades. Such children are being brought out of the closets and being mainstreamed into their rightful places in society. Acceptance of the handicapped in social and educational settings, even though mandated by law, is being accomplished through better understanding by the community and through the development of community resources to support this type of handicapped individual. For the first time in history, the developmentally disabled child is taking his rightful place in society as an individual human being.

FETAL ALCOHOL SYNDROME

The effect of alcohol in causing defects in children born to mothers who are chronic alcoholics has been known for many centuries. It has only been in recent years, since 1973 to be exact, that a specific fetal alcohol syndrome has been reported and identified as occurring in children born to chronic alcoholic mothers.

In the 1700s the British government made gin a legal beverage without taxation in an effort to raise grain prices. This resulted in what has been known as the "gin epidemic," resulting in rather serious consequences. In 1751 Henry Fielding wrote, "Who is conceived in gin, with the poisonous distillations of which it is nourished, both in the womb and at the breast, will be malformed.'' In the latter part of the 1700s the British government ended the taxation relief, thus ending this acute social problem as well.

Children with the alcohol syndrome have a pattern of defects which include prenatal and postnatal growth deficiency, small head size, mental retardation, and delayed growth and development. Certain facial abnormalities, particularly a small jaw (micrognathia), droopy eyelids, thin upper lips, and a poorly formed upper jaw, are frequently noted. It is not uncommon to find cardiac defects, usually a defect in the septum of the heart, and decreased range of motion in extremities is frequently reported. This group of children show the full-blown classic fetal alcohol syndrome. There is evidence today that less serious defects occur. Some children not showing the full-blown syndrome may present with minor problems of hyperactivity, decreased learning ability, small stature, and some behavioral problems. A large number of these mildly affected children appear to be able to grow out of their difficulties with proper stimulation and education programs.

The more severely affected children often fail to thrive in terms of survival, adaptation to life after being born, and general physical growth. Mental deficiency is of varying severity and is probably the most serious consequence being related to the amount of brain damage apparently caused by the alcohol.

The exact mechanism of damage is unknown but is thought to be due specifically to the alcohol or to a metabolic breakdown product of alcohol transmitted from the mother to the fetus through the placenta. It does not appear to be due to malnutrition, although this can occur in chronic alcoholics. The defects seen in the children are not similar to those seen in severe malnutrition; indeed, in the few cases that have been monitored, malnutrition does not appear to play a role in the production of birth defects. The range of damage that exists is probably quite broad, and considerable study still remains to be done to delineate this entity. One thing is certain, that those with severe damage continue to show delayed growth and failure to thrive.

Perhaps the first question to ask is, ''How much drinking is harmful?'' At present, it is not known. Studies to date indicate that a pregnant woman is at risk if she drinks three or more ounces of absolute alcohol daily (100% alcohol), which would be equivalent to six ounces of 100 proof alcohol. This is equivalent to about six to eight average-size drinks. The current recommendation from the U.S. Department of Health, Education, and Welfare, the Alcohol and Drug Abuse Bureau is that pregnant women should drink no more than one ounce of absolute alcohol per day which is the equivalent of two mixed drinks containing about one ounce of liquor each, or two five-ounce glasses of wine, or two twelve-ounce cans of beer. Saving up drinks is not permitted. Two drinks per day means just that. Saving up drinks through the week and having six or eight on a Saturday night party could be dangerous to a baby's health.

At the present time, there is not enough information to set specific guidelines. The best advice that can be given to women who are pregnant or contemplating pregnancy is that they do all things in moderation and that they be moderate in their drinking habits. If there are further specific concerns, it is advisable to discuss them with a health professional. Additional information is available from the U.S. Department of Health, Education, and Welfare. The address is listed in Appendix 2.

SMOKING EFFECTS ON NEWBORNS

Unfortunately, the literature dealing with the effects of smoking during pregnancy, in many instances, appears to be extremely biased, both pro and con.

One effect has become quite clear in recent years: mothers who are heavy smokers, smoking one pack or more of cigarettes per day, have a higher incidence of children with a low birthweight for the state of gestation. We classify this child as one born at "low weight for date of gestation." These children are usually delivered at their normal due date of 40 weeks gestation, but they will frequently weigh only 4 to 5 pounds instead of the usual 6 to 7½ pounds.

Although the exact cause of this difficulty is not fully understood at this time, it is felt that it is either related to the direct effect of nicotine on the uterine vessels, causing a decrease in the blood supply to the uterus, or to an effect of the carbon monoxide content of the inhaled cigarette smoke. The most likely culprit is the carbon monoxide, as there is an increase of blood carboxyhemoglobin levels (hemoglobin with carbon monoxide attached rather than oxygen) with values averaging 7% to 8% in smoking women as compared to 1% in nonsmoking women.

A Canadian Collaborative Project has definitely pointed to a greater risk of fetal and perinatal death in infants of women who smoke more than one pack of cigarettes per day. In this group of women, perinatal mortality (death about the time of delivery) was 33.4 infant deaths per 1000 births compared with 23.3 deaths per 1000 births for nonsmokers. In this category of smoking mothers, the fetal deaths were largely attributed to unknown causes and to anoxia, while the neonatal deaths, those occurring right after birth, were attributed chiefly to prematurity and respiratory problems.

In the Canadian studies there was, however, less smoking-associated risk for women who were young, on their first or second pregnancy, and who were private patients from a higher socioeconomic stratum. The exact cause of this difference has not yet been described.

Some long-term follow-up studies of low-birthweight children indicate that many have an increased incidence of mild mental retardation, hyperactivity, behavioral difficulties, and coordination problems. This association has been questioned by other studies which report no long-term effects of maternal smoking on physical growth and intellectual development. There has been a general lack of control of significant variables in investigating these populations, making conclusions difficult. Unfortunately, many studies do not differentiate as to specific causes of the low-birthweight-for-date infants. Several of the causes are not related to smoking. Further investigation needs to be accomplished.

Recent studies released from the U.S. Collaborative Perinatal Project indicate that there may be a negative effect of smoking that continues even if women quit before pregnancy. This study would indicate that there are increased placental abnormalities related to past smoking as well as current smoking. Confirmation of these data must still be obtained.

Because of the vast differences in people and their smoking habits, whether they are puffers or inhalers, the type of cigarette they smoke, and the amount of filter that is used, it is difficult at this time to determine just how damaging smoking might be in any one individual. Here again, we recommend moderation and suggest that women who are heavy smokers, if they are planning to conceive or become pregnant, should discuss this in detail with their physicians.

PRENATAL DIAGNOSIS BY AMNIOCENTESIS

Amniocentesis is a diagnostic technique that has become available in the past few years. It permits prenatal diagnosis of certain genetic, chromosomal, and neural tube defects. Through the use of this test, many of the inborn errors of metabolism, the chromosomal defects, and most of the defects in the neural tube, eg, spina bifida, meningomyelocele, can be diagnosed in utero.

Many thousands of these procedures have been carried out in the early part of the second trimester of pregnancy, and when done properly in well-controlled clinics, it is virtually free from risk and gives a high reliability approaching 96%.

A National Institute of Child Health and Human Development study involved over 1000 mothers in a group having an amniocentesis during the second trimester and a control group of a similar number. The two groups showed no significant difference in fetal loss, adverse occurrences during pregnancy, premature live births, condition of the newborn, or development up to age one year.

Fetal loss due to spontaneous abortion (a medical term for miscarriage in the first few months) was virtually identical in the two groups.

They were unable to report any fetal loss directly related to the amniocentesis. It is true there have been some rare difficulties reported, but these are extremely minor; the safety appears to be beyond question.

Amniocentesis is usually performed between the fifteenth and sixteenth weeks of gestation. The reason for choosing this time is that it is necessary to wait until about the fifteenth week before there is adequate amniotic fluid to permit a safe procedure. At the tenth week of gestation there is only 30 to 40 ml of amniotic fluid, while at the fifteenth week the amount increases to about 350 ml.

The procedure is frequently preceded by an ultrasound (radiosound) examination to locate the position of the fetal head and the placenta. After these are located and the doctor carefully examines the patient, a local anesthetic is injected in the skin, a needle inserted into the uterus, and 10 to 20 cc of fluid is withdrawn (Figure 8-1).

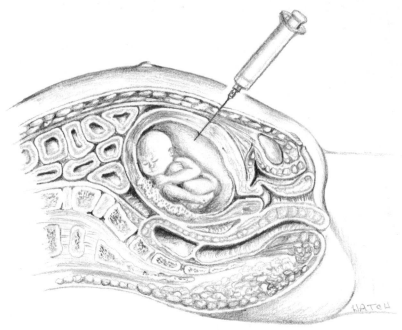

Figure 8-1 Technique of amniocentesis. The needle is inserted into the amniotic cavity and fluid removed.

This fluid contains cells, which are then available for culture and can be examined in the biochemical laboratory for chemical substances diagnostic of certain diseases. The amniotic cells, which come from the baby, not the mother, are placed in tissue culture media and permitted to grow in incubators in the laboratory. Routine chromosome studies are performed on these cells to determine if there are any chromosomal abnormalities present in the baby (Figure 8-2).

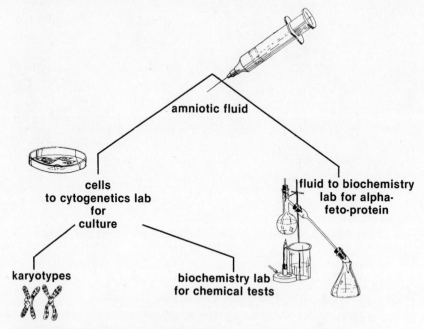

Figure 8-2 Processing of amniotic fluid.

The fluid is sent to the biochemical laboratory where it is examined to determine the amount of alpha-feto-protein present. Alpha-feto-protein is a substance produced within the central nervous system in the developing embryo. If there is a defect in the development of the neural tube, as occurs in most cases of spina bifida and meningomyelocele, there is an increased amount of this substance present in the amniotic fluid. If this is elevated, an attempt can be made to establish further the diagnosis of a neural tube defect using ultrasound and, in some cases, a repeat amniocentesis.

After the cells are cultured, two things can be done. A certain group of cells are utilized to perform and make karyograms to look at the chromosome structure of the infant. Other cells can be used for chemical determinations to search for the absence or excess of enzymes that are characteristic or diagnostic of one of the inborn errors of metabolism.

The karyograms can tell many things. They establish the sex of a child; contrary to all the old wives' tales, this is the only sure way. They provide evidence by showing extra chromosomes, as in Down syndrome, or an absent chromosome, as in Turner syndrome. It is also possible to find small deletions or additions to chromosomes or translocations (which occur when a chromosome in whole or part adheres to one of the other chromosomes). Enlarged photographs can be analyzed by karyotyping, as described in Chapter 9.

It is necessary to understand that karyotypes cannot look at individual genes. Genes are extremely small microscopic particles which cannot be seen with the aid of the usual microscopic techniques we have today, so the presence or absence of any specific genes cannot be determined by this technique. This procedure looks at the gross chromosome structure only.

There are several indications for advising a pregnant woman in her early pregnancy about the availability of an amniocentesis. Amniocentesis should be discussed in depth between a physician and his patient as to whether the procedure is advisable under certain situations. The following indications call for consideration of an amniocentesis:

1. Early pregnancy at age 35 or over.
2. A woman having a previous child with a trisomy, eg, Down syndrome; trisomy-13, 18.
3. Either parent known to carry a chromosomal translocation.
4. Any families at risk for X-linked (sex-linked) recessive disorders such as Duchenne muscular dystrophy.
5. Families at risk for an autosomal recessive disorder, known to be detectable in utero by a chemical examination, such as Tay-Sachs disease.
6. Any parents having had a previous child with anencephaly, meningomyelocele, or other neural tube defect (risk of recurrence in these couples approximates 5% to 7%).

The most frequent indication and the majority of people seeking counseling concerning amniocentesis are the older mothers of age 35 or over.

A few pitfalls, arising infrequently in prenatal diagnosis, make it difficult to arrive at a firm diagnosis. They include mosaicism, a condition where part of the person's cells might have a chromosomal defect and the other part does not. It is possible that only the normal cells will be found in a single culture of amniotic cells, and a normal karyotype does not necessarily rule out a mosaicism. These circumstances, however, are extremely rare. In years past, it was difficult to find small translocations, but with the availability of new laboratory techniques, these should all be found.

Culturing amniotic fluid cells takes approximately three weeks to permit the cells to grow and divide so that the chromosome structures can be determined during the process of division.

Also, this period of time permits the proliferation and growth of cells until sufficient numbers are obtained to permit certain specific biochemical tests to be done to determine the presence or absence of certain enzymes. These enzyme tests are not performed on all amniocenteses; they are done only when there is a family history suggestive of an inborn error of metabolism.

Many types of inborn errors of metabolism can be determined at the present time. This number is increasing and as biochemical expertise improves, more of these metabolic difficulties will be diagnosed. Individually, these diseases are quite rare; but collectively, they occur in about one in every 5000 to 8000 live births. These are usually diseases which result from an inherited disorder due to a gene defect.

Prenatal diagnosis is not generally undertaken for this type of biochemical abnormality unless the parents have already had one child with this type of defect or unless there is a strong family history and testing of the parents has indicated that both are carriers of this disease. In all cases, specific genetic counseling should be undertaken by the parents before pursuing this type of diagnostic regimen.

Among the X-linked or sex-linked genetic diseases that can be detected by finding deficiency of an enzyme in cultures of the amniotic cells are Fabry disease, Hunter syndrome, and the Lesch-Nyhan syndromes. Unfortunately, many X-linked diseases cannot be detected prenatally because the abnormality does not manifest itself as an abnormal enzyme and frequently will not create the disease problem until later life. These include such diseases as Duchenne muscular dystrophy, hemophilia, Menke syndrome, and several immunodeficiency diseases. In disease entities that are X-linked and in which the disorder is recessive, the disease will become apparent in 50% of all male fetuses if the mother is a carrier. In situations where it is necessary to avoid any chance of propagation of this disease by aborting all males, one-half of those aborted will be affected and one-half will be unaffected.

There are other inborn errors of metabolism which are usually associated with the autosome and are not sex-linked. These diseases involve abnormalities of carbohydrate, amino acid, and lipid metabolism. All these diseases apparently involve a gene mutation that prohibits the production of proper enzyme that is essential in a portion of the metabolic cycle in the body. Diseases of lipid metabolism include the gangliosidoses, which include pseudo-Hurler syndrome, Tay-Sachs disease, Sandhoff disease, Gaucher disease, and metachromatic leukodystrophy.

In certain diseases of carbohydrate metabolism, the glycogen storage disease such as Pompe galactosemia, and fucosidosis can be detected. Galactosemia, when detected either prenatally or immediately after birth, can be treated if a restricted diet is started early in life. The mucopolysaccharide diseases occur in about one in 25,000 live births in the United

States, producing approximately 250 cases per year of children with these various diseases. All these are associated with an accumulation of mucopolysaccharides in various tissues of the body.

Hurler disease, an autosomal recessive, and Hunter disease, which is X-linked, can both be detected in utero through special techniques which utilize the incorporation of radioactive materials in the cells being cultured.

The disorders of the amino acid metabolism occur in about one in 3000 live births overall. The most common is PKU (phenylketonuria) which occurs in about one in 10,000 to 12,000 live births. Unfortunately, it is impossible at this time to detect the presence of PKU prenatally, as it is necessary that the infant have an intake of specific proteins found principally in milk. A milk intake for 12 to 24 hours is necessary before blood or urine levels can evidence abnormal quantities of phenylalanine. For this reason, it is important that newborn babies have a PKU test after 12 to 24 hours of milk feedings. In the event that for any reason there is a failure to have the test done, it should be performed within a few days and then repeated between two and four weeks. Only if both these tests are completed is it possible to detect adequately all the cases of PKU which will occur in the United States.

There are a number of other very rare diseases such as the Lesch-Nyhan syndrome, the I-cell disease, lysosomal acid phosphatase deficiency, and xeroderma pigmentosa which can also be detected in utero. It is anticipated that in the future, as enzymatic and biochemical pathways become better known, many other rare but severely debilitating diseases can be detected in utero, and preventive measures or treatment programs can be instituted.

Cystic fibrosis is probably one of the most common of the severe genetic diseases. It occurs once in every 2500 live births. At the present time, prenatal diagnosis of this entity is impossible as we do not know the biochemical defect occurring in these children. Considerable work is being done attempting to uncover the biochemistry of this rather severe disease.

Central nervous system malformations presenting as severe neural tube defects such as anencephaly, meningomyelocele, and spina bifida occur in one of every 200 to 2000 live births. This appears to be increased in Wales and in certain parts of Ireland; the exact cause for this is unknown. In these cases, as mentioned previously, the alpha-feto-protein levels increase during the second trimester of pregnancy. The reliability of detection approximates 85% to 90%. In cases of anencephaly or the absence of the major part of the brain, the cerebrum, there is also an increase in the alpha-feto-protein level. This entity can be detected and can usually be confirmed by an ultrasound examination. It is usually customary to monitor a pregnant woman only after she has had one affected child. The monitor is done by ultrasonography, using ultrasound to determine the size of the baby's head. In many cases, it is also possible to detect spina bifida if it is present and protruding as a meningomyelocele.

The ability to detect some of the more severe hemoglobinopathies such as sickle cell disease and thalassemia is limited at this time. Approximately 8% of the blacks in the United States today are heterozygous or carry the gene for sickle cell disease without showing it. Approximately one in 625 live births in the black population are children homozygous for sickle cell anemia, which means the severe manifestation of this disease. The ability to detect sickle cell disease in utero is limited because it is necessary to secure an actual blood sample of the baby's blood to make this diagnosis.

Techniques are being developed in using a fetoscope, an instrument inserted into the uterus to look at the fetus. (This is similar to what the doctor does as he looks into the bladder during cystoscopy or down into the lungs during bronchoscopy.) The use of fetoscopy is increasing at the present time and is useful to help in diagnosis and treatment of certain rare disease problems. Perhaps in the future it will be possible to obtain blood from the fetus by doing a venipuncture of one of the umbilical veins through the fetoscope. This procedure is not readily available; if it appears to be indicated, it should be discussed with an obstetrician.

There are several other reasons for doing amniotic fluid examinations, usually later in pregnancy. One of these is Rh incompatibility where sensitization has occurred in the mother. The level of bilirubin is determined to give an index as to the rapidity or severity of disease which might be occurring in the infant.

Lecithin/sphingomyelin ratios are also determined late in pregnancy as these appear to give an index of the maturity of the fetal lungs. Particularly in cases of diabetes or other conditions where it may be necessary to try to induce labor early, an L/S determination may be done to see if the lungs are mature enough to support the infant outside the uterus.

After the diagnoses are performed, what are their values? Reports indicate that there are positive findings in approximately 2.2% of the mothers age 35 to 39, 3.4% in those over age 40, and approximately 5% in those over 44. The probable overall percentage today (since there is an increase in younger women requesting amniocentesis because of an abnormal family history) would indicate approximately 2% to 3% positive findings.

The decision to terminate the pregnancy if there is an abnormal child in the uterus is one that must rest with the parents. In order to arrive at a reasonable decision, the parents involved should discuss this in depth with their physician, with a genetic counselor, if available, and with their religious leader if there are ethical problems. The decision to terminate pregnancy should be arrived at after a careful consideration of all these concerns. It is not a decision that should be reached by a physician, either for or against such a termination, but one that can only be reached by both parents after proper counseling and advice.

A frequently asked question is, "Should I have an amniocentesis performed even though I know I will not have this pregnancy terminated no matter what the outcome of the test might be?" It has been our experience that there are some women who desire to have the test done simply because of the relief they feel by knowing that it is a normal pregnancy 95% to 98% of the time. In a few cases, these parents even have felt some relief when they know that it is another Down child. The great enigma of not knowing appears to be an extremely frustrating thing to most people.

Information as to counseling centers can be obtained from the National Foundation March of Dimes. Their address is listed in Appendix 2, "Services for Handicapped Children and Their Families."

9 Genetics

Genetics, stated very simply, is the scientific study of inheritance. It is the science dealing with inherited attributes—good, bad, and indifferent —passed from a mother and a father to their child. The inherited characteristics passed on to each succeeding generation was received from the preceding generation of parents. Thus, there is a continuum of inheritance patterns from generation to generation. In the process of gene selection, however, certain genetic characteristics may be lost as the germ cells divide, and new characteristics are added to the gene pool of any one individual from the other member of a mating. A spontaneous change in the chemical structure of a gene with a resulting new strain of gene is called a mutation. Mutations may be good or bad. They may cause changes that are incompatible with survival, or they may act to improve the species.

Discussion and writings on genetics are as old as history. Even in the early ages of time, historians recorded the transmission of family characteristics and traits; these traits were noted "to make the son look like unto the father." The ancient writings of Egypt, Greece, and the Hebrews give us information that these ancient cultures had limited, but basic, knowledge of genetic transmission in both humans and animals. It was for this reason that the intermarriage of close family members was either forbidden or at least avoided in most instances.

Avoidance was not always practiced in some of the royal houses of Egypt and the aristocracy and royal lineages of Europe. The practices in these families tended to ignore these theologic or philosophic warnings. A practice of genetic inbreeding resulted, which was accomplished principally for the purpose of maintaining a social stratum and preserving the "purity of the blood lines."

Inbreeding in these families did result in the development of an increased incidence of recessive genetic disease. The most classic case of this is hemophilia, "the royal disease." This disease became prominent in some of the royal houses of Europe during the eighteenth and nineteenth centuries. Hemophilia is a recessive, sex-linked genetic disease occurring almost always in males.

The first scientific reports on heritability were published by Gregor Mendel in about 1860. He reported certain basic laws of inheritance of dominant and recessive transmission which remain unchallenged. Today, we call this type of heritability "mendelian" and classify it as following the "mendelian law."

The scientific study of genetics, unfortunately, then entered a 40-year period of hibernation as Mendel's work was almost forgotten until the early 1900s when other scientists and researchers rediscovered and applied his work. Genetics has progressed rapidly since that time and is undergoing almost explosive research at the present time.

Although the concept of the existence of human chromosomes was reported as early as the 1870s, it was not until 1956 that the human chromosome number was correctly and accurately described. Human cells contain 46 chromosomes, in 23 pairs. Of these, 22 pairs or 44 chromosomes are called autosomes. The sex chromosomes make up the other pair. The sex chromosomes are of two types, the X and the Y chromosomes. Human females have two X chromosomes (Figure 9-1) and the male, an X and a Y chromosome (Figure 9-2). The size and shape of the two X chromosomes in the female are the same. In the male, the X and Y chromosomes are of different size, the Y being much smaller and containing only a very limited amount of genetic material.

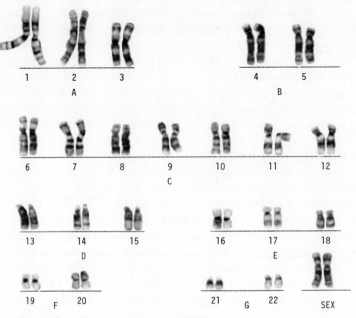

Figure 9-1 Normal female karyotype–46XX.

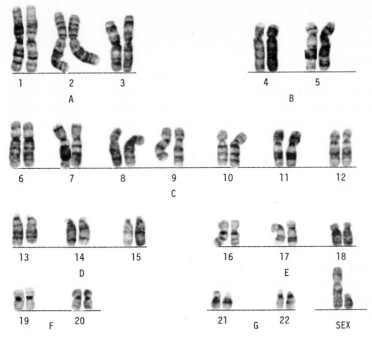

Figure 9-2 Normal male karyotype–46XY.

One member of each pair of chromosomes, both the autosomes and the sex chromosomes, is derived from the father, and the other member of the pair is derived from the mother. The infant, therefore, receives 50% of his genetic complement from his father and 50% from his mother.

All the cells in the body, with the exception of the gametes, or sex cells, contain the diploid complement of 46 chromosomes, except in those individuals with one of the gross chromosomal abnormalities to be described. The gametic cells, the egg in the female and the sperm in the male, have only one member of each chromosome pair; therefore, they have only 23 chromosomes. This leads to the diploid number of 46 after fertilization occurs.

Chromosomes are composed of deoxyribonucleic acid (DNA), whose chemical structure was only recently described. The DNA content in each nucleus in the body is quantitatively and qualitatively identical in any one individual, even though different types of cells are of different size, shape, and perform different functions within the body.

Modern medical genetics is progressing extremely rapidly, and information published in texts today will be outmoded almost before leaving the publisher. It is a field only 20 years young, and yet it has improved the identification and understanding of many disease processes. As new techniques become available in future years, it is anticipated that it will be possible to diagnose even more genetic abnormalities. Future studies of the chromosomes, the genetically endowed chemical behavior of cells grown in tissue culture, and the inheritability of diseases will lead to better understanding and improved therapy of many of the diseases of man.

The first chromosomal abnormality was described in 1959 when it was noted that individuals with Down syndrome had an extra chromosome—a complement of 47 chromosomes in all their cells. This was noted to be an extra No. 21 chromosome, hence, this syndrome has been called trisomy-21. (See Chapter 12 on Down Syndrome, and Figure 12-1.)

Also in 1959, Turner and Klinefelter syndromes were equated with a chromosomal abnormality. In these cases, the abnormality involved the sex chromosomes. Females with Turner syndrome have only one X chromosome, or a total complement of 45 chromosomes, missing one of the two X chromosomes. Klinefelter syndrome manifests an extra X chromosome in the male. These males have a chromosome count of 47 with an XXY sex chromosome. Both syndromes are discussed in Chapter 11. See Figures 11-2 and 11-3.

Progress during the years from 1959 to 1965 was rapid, and there were increasing reports of many different types of gross chromosomal abnormalities. These were described as involving either extra chromosomes or absent chromosomes. Next, conditions were described in which there was either an addition or a loss of a part of a chromosome. The first such deletion reported was the cri du chat syndrome. Children with this difficulty are born missing a small portion of the No. 5 chromosome. This condition causes severe mental and motor retardation. (See Figure 11-1.)

Only since 1970 have staining techniques made it possible to positively identify each individual chromosome. Prior to 1970, the chromosomes stained as one color, and though it was possible to divide them into groups of a similar size and shape, the identification of each one was not possible. With the advent in 1970 of a new staining technique called G-banding, all 46 individual chromosomes could be identified by distinctive banding patterns.

Chromosomes can be seen under the light microscope at a magnification of about 1000X. Individual genes cannot be seen. Genes are extremely small molecular structures consisting of localized sequences of DNA specifying one cellular function only; there are many hundreds to thousands of genes located on each chromosome. Genes might be viewed as the small individual beads making up a compact necklace, the chromosome. Only recently have genes been described and photographed under extremely high magnification with the electron microscope. At the present state of our knowledge, it is not possible to identify abnormal genes by studying a karyotype. Only the gross, large structures, the chromosomes, can be identified and examined with today's microscopic technology.

KARYOTYPING AND MAPPING

The chromosomal disorders in man are unique in that they lend themselves to direct laboratory analysis by a method called chromosome karyotyping, which is the finished product of chromosome studies. In this study, representative samples of chromosomes are photographed and enlargements are printed. The chromosomes are then individually cut out and pasted on a chart after each of the individual 46 chromosomes are identified. This cutout is called a karyotype.

In 1960, a group of world geneticists meeting at a convention in Denver agreed upon the numbering sequence of the chromosomes. The numbering depends upon the size and shape of the chromosome and the location of the centromere (the narrowed portion of each chromosome). The largest chromosome was labeled No. 1 and the smallest No. 22. The No. 23 pair are the X and Y, or the sex, chromosomes.

Karyotyping can be accomplished from several different kinds of tissue, provided the tissue is alive and capable of growing and dividing. The major sources of tissues for karyotypes are either the white blood cells obtained from a blood specimen or fibroblasts secured from a skin biopsy and allowed to grow in a special tissue culture. Occasionally, bone marrow cells or tissue from other organs are used in culture preparations.

Blood is the most frequently used source, as it is possible to accomplish growth rapidly, and a finished karyotype can be made available within five to seven days in urgent cases. The blood cells used are the white blood cells, the lymphocytes, which are permitted to grow in a special culture medium for three days after their growth is stimulated by phytohemagglutinin. After about 72 hours, colchicine is added to the culture medium, arresting the growth of the cells in a cell division stage known as metaphase. In the metaphase the chromosomes are most compact and lend themselves most readily to examination under the microscope. These cells are then harvested, spread on microscope slides, dried, stained, and examined through the microscope. Photographs are taken and the karyotype made; this is a rather lengthy and time-consuming process.

Cells grown from tissue sources other than blood, eg, a skin biopsy, require a much longer time to accomplish growth and division of cells. Most fibroblast cultures from skin biopsies will require three to six weeks before there is sufficient growth of the cells to harvest them and to make the karyotype.

In looking at certain types of disease, it is important to try to determine the location of specific genes on a definite chromosome. This chromosome mapping is being accomplished slowly and arduously with the identification of specific locations, or loci, where these individual genes are located. These loci have been identified for well over 100 different specific genes at the present time, and new gene locations are being reported frequently.

The amount of genetic disease occurring in the United States today is extensive and is not limited to gross chromosomal abnormalities or rare diseases. More than 22 million individuals in the United States either have or will develop a disease having a strong genetic component. At the present time, more than 2800 individual genetic diseases have been identified and cataloged. (See V.A. McKusick in Appendix 3.) More genetic diseases are being added, and it is expected that this list will continue to grow. In many cases, such diseases as diabetes and hypertension are being relegated to their proper positions as genetic.

GENETIC DISEASES

Genetic diseases involve a significant financial burden, as 25% to 50% of all admissions to major children's hospitals in the United States have a clearly defined or strong genetic component in the illness. It can be seen that inherited disease inflicts a severe penalty, both in suffering and in the cost of health care. Careful genetic counseling and advice can help to reduce the incidence of many of these illnesses.

Genetic disease can be classified into three general categories: 1) gross chromosomal abnormalities, eg, Down syndrome; 2) monogenic diseases, involving only one gene. These diseases may have either a recessive or dominant transmission, eg, PKU; and 3) polygenic disorders —where there is an involvement of more than one, sometimes many, genes, eg, diabetes, hypertension, neural tube defects.

In discussing genetic diseases and patterns of inheritance, certain terminology should be understood:

Allele   Genes that are on the same locus of the same pair of chromosomes are alleles. They are concerned with the same category of information, though perhaps in a somewhat different fashion. For example, genes of blood groups A, B, and O are alleles.

Homozygous   A person with a pair of identical alleles at a given location on a pair of chromosomes is said to be homozygous. If both alleles are abnormal, the disease is expressed, eg, PKU.

Heterozygous   A person with two different alleles at a single locus on a pair of chromosomes is heterozygous. If the gene is dominant and abnormal, the disease is expressed, eg, Duchenne muscular dystrophy. If the gene is recessive, the disease is not expressed, eg, a female carrier for hemophilia.

Karyotype   The chromosome complement arranged and analyzed according to size and banding patterns is a karyotype.

Trisomy This is a condition where the total number of chromosomes equals 47 with a triple dose in one of the chromosomes instead of the usual pair.

Autosomal trisomy This occurs when there is a triple dose of one of the autosomes, eg, Down–Trisomy-21.

Sex chromosome trisomy This occurs when there are three sex chromosomes, eg, XXX, XXY, XYY.

Monosomy Monosomy occurs when one chromosome is missing and the complement is 45 chromosomes. The missing chromosome might be an autosome or one of the sex chromosomes. Autosomal monosomy appears to be incompatible with life, as these conditions are only found in material obtained from miscarriages. A monosomic abnormality of the sex chromosomes results in a Turner syndrome, or an XO karyotype.

CHROMOSOMAL ABNORMALITIES

Chromosomal aberrations may be due either to abnormal numbers of chromosomes, *aneuploidies,* or to structural abnormalities involving one or more of the chromosomes. Aneuploidies may involve all the cells of the individual or they may be *mosaic*—a condition where the individual has two to more cell lines, at least one of which is abnormal.

In mosaic disease, the person will have cells of two different, but related, genetic makeups. These situations occur when there is an abnormal cell division early after fertilization, with the production of two cell lines. One cell line perhaps containing 46 chromosomes and the other cell line 45 or 47 chromosomes. Many times, people with mosaic disease are not as severely affected as their counterparts with a nonmosaic chromosome abnormality. Careful studies are necessary in diagnosing and counseling people with these disorders.

The incidence of aneuploidies in newborns is quite high, with reports showing the incidence from 0.3% to 0.7%, or a frequency of about one in 150 to 300 newborns. The most common abnormalities are Down syndrome with a frequency of 1:720; Turner syndrome (XO), 1:5000; trisomy-13, 1:7000 to 12,000; trisomy-18, 1:3000 to 10,000; and Klinefelter syndrome, 1:800.

The incidence of aneuploidies, though high in newborns, is even higher during prenatal life and results in frequent spontaneous abortions (miscarriages). Studies have indicated that from 25% to 60% of spontaneous abortions have chromosomal abnormalities, most often an aneuploidy. It is quite possible that this incidence is low if all spontaneous abortions examined were to include the extremely early fetal loss which might occur at the time when the mother is not quite sure she is pregnant. All told, it is estimated that between 2.5% and 10% of all conceptuses have a chromosomal abnormality.

Women having recurrent spontaneous abortions, particularly those with three or more, should seek genetic counseling to determine the advisability of having karyotypes done on both parents to determine if some abnormal chromosome pattern might exist in the parents themselves.

Chromosomal studies of aborted material, where available, should also be considered in women having recurrent spontaneous abortions, as the recurrence risk of having another chromosomal abnormality can be greater than in the general population if an aneuploidy is present in the aborted specimen.

When a spontaneous abortion occurs with the passage of a formed embryo, the obstetrician or the pathologist should, if at all possible, examine the specimen carefully to determine if there is any obvious defect. This is particularly true with cases of neural tube disorders such as spina bifida, anencephaly, or meningomyelocele. The recurrence risk of having a subsequent child with a neural tube defect in future pregnancies is about 5%. Usually this disorder can be diagnosed prenatally by means of amniocentesis and ultrasound techniques. (Amniocentesis was discussed at the end of Chapter 8.)

The story of chromosome abnormalities becomes more complicated when translocation and mosaicism are introduced. Translocations imply the transfer of a portion of one chromosome to another chromosome. Figure 9-3 illustrates a translocation of a portion of one of the No. 14 chromosomes to one of the No. 6 chromosomes. In this particular individual, the translocation is "balanced" in that there is no loss of genetic material. This individual is perfectly normal. The major difficulty encountered by people with translocations if the translocations are balanced, is that there is difficulty in their having children because abnormal sperm or eggs are being produced. Translocations can occur in many different chromosomes and can account for abnormal chromosome structures in offspring. Careful genetic counseling is required in each individual case.

In the population at large, balanced translocations occur in about 1.9 per 1000 live births, and unbalanced translocations occur in about one in every 2000 live births. The unbalanced translocation almost invariably causes serious birth defects or mental retardation. Even small deletions can cause serious mental retardation frequently accompanied by abnormal physical development.

The majority of chromosomal abnormalities seen are not transmitted from the parents to the affected child but occur as a result of an abnormal division occurring either in the gametes as they are developing or in the fertilized egg during the process of its early division. In cases of translocation, in deletion or addition of chromosomes, and in mosaic disease, karyotyping of the parents is necessary to determine if there is an inherited condition which could be transmitted to future offspring.

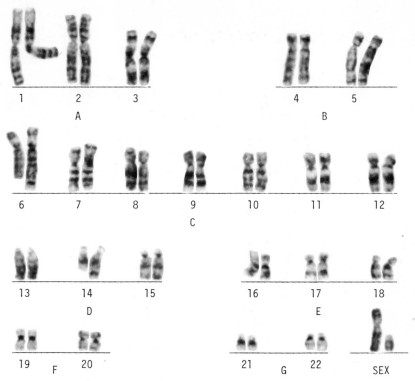

Figure 9-3 Karyotype showing a 6:14 translocation.

MONOGENIC DISEASE

Monogenic disorders are caused by the presence of a single abnormal gene. Within our genetic makeup, all of us have from five to ten "bad" genes; if mated with a person carrying a similar abnormal gene, a specific disease will occur in the offspring. Over 2800 disorders of this type have been recognized and are presently cataloged. These disorders can be caused by dominant genes or recessive genes. They might involve the autosomes or the sex chromosomes, particularly the X chromosome. To date, over 107 different genes have been identified as being present on the X chromosome. This number will continue to grow as research progresses.

In autosomal dominant genetic diseases, the gene causing the disease dominates its partner on the other chromosome of the pair (Figure 9-4). In dominant conditions, it is necessary to have only one abnormal gene to produce disease. In these situations, all persons carrying the gene will show the trait (it might be a disease or it might be genes producing certain physical traits, eg, brown eyes are dominant over blue eyes).

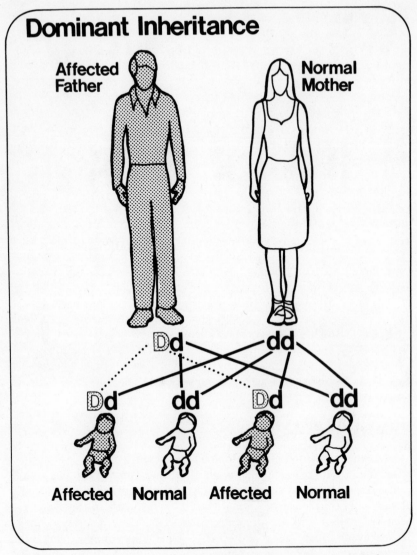

Dominant Inheritance

Affected Father

Normal Mother

Dd   dd

Dd   dd   Dd   dd

Affected   Normal   Affected   Normal

Figure 9-4 Dominant inheritance—One affected parent has a single faulty gene (D) which *dominates* its normal counterpart (d). Each child has a 50% chance of inheriting the faulty gene from the affected parent. Adapted from: The New Human Genetics. DHEW Publ. No. (NIH) 76-662.

In children produced by people with a dominant gene, 50% of the offspring can receive the gene and the autosomal dominant trait will be manifest. Therefore, in a conception, there is a 50/50 chance of a child receiving the abnormal gene and a 50/50 chance that the child will receive the normal gene. This same 50/50 chance holds for all future conceptions.

The fact that a parent has a dominant disease and has produced either several children free of the disease or several children with the disease does not change these statistics on the next pregnancy. The chances will still be 50/50 that the child will receive the gene for this dominant trait.

Marriages between first cousins make it much more likely that there will be a sharing of similar harmful genes, and it is for this reason that first-cousin marriages are not usually advised.

The severity of any disease caused by the presence of an abnormal gene can vary widely from individual to individual. In other words, there is variability in the "expression" that this gene makes in the production of any abnormalities. Thus there can be a lot of variation from one individual to another and from one generation to another in autosomal dominant disease.

In these dominant diseases, most individuals have only one single abnormal gene and are therefore heterozygous. In rare situations where both parents are affected with this dominant trait, children of this couple can receive two affected, or abnormal, genes and be homozygous. In most cases, the severity of dominant disease in the homozygous state is higher and the disability much greater.

Autosomal dominant disease is not always congenital, that is, not always manifest at birth. Probably some of the most widespread dominant genetic diseases in the country today are certain types of familial hypercholesterolemia; manifestations of this disease do not become apparent until middle age. Laboratory evidence of the disease can be found in younger children by testing for excessive quantities of cholesterol in their blood.

Huntington chorea, another dominant disease, does not manifest itself until about age 50. Gardner syndrome, a dominant genetic condition which causes polyps to form in the colon with a high propensity for malignancy, and certain cases of autosomal dominant breast cancer have been identified. In these cases, knowledge about the dominant genetic nature of the disease will forewarn parents and permit them to have their children undergo careful evaluation to prevent, where possible, the development of severe disease, or allow the institution of therapy early in the course of the illness.

On occasion, a dominant disorder occurs where there is no family history suggesting a disease. This is particularly true in achondroplastic dwarfism. In this disease, new mutations are the most frequent cause of the production of an achondroplastic child.

Such dominant disorders as neurofibromatosis and tuberous sclerosis may present in a child where the parents show minimal symptoms of the disease entity. In both these conditions, it is sometimes necessary to search diligently in the parent for physical findings consistent with these diseases.

A list of autosomal dominant diseases follows:

Marfan syndrome
von Recklinghausen disease (neurofibromatosis)
Huntington chorea
polycystic kidney disease
Conradi disease
polysyndactyly
Sticker syndrome
Holt-Oram syndrome
certain types of hyperlipoproteinemia

Certain dominant disorders appear to occur more frequently in men than women. These conditions are sex-linked, and the dominant gene appears to be carried on the X chromosome. Gout, baldness, and hemophilia occurring in men are frequent examples of dominant traits expressed principally in males.

X-linked, or sex-linked, dominant disorders are relatively uncommon. These are characterized by involvement in each generation with the ratio of the affected females to males being 2:1. There is an absence of male-to-male transmission, and males are usually more severely affected than females. In these situations, there are no unaffected carriers, as individuals with only one abnormal gene will manifest the disease.

Each daughter and each son of an affected woman would have a 50% chance of having the disorder. None of the sons of an affected male would have the disease, but all his daughters would have the disorder.

X-linked dominant disorders are:

pseudohypoparathyroidism
  (Albright hereditary osteodystrophy)
focal dermal hypoplasia
phosphate diabetes

In many cases there is an interplay with environmental factors that modify the expression of the genetic abnormality. They may cause an early or delayed precipitation of the disease, or they may increase or decrease the expression of the disease. Unfortunately, things are not always clearcut and can be changed by modifying the environment. Such modification occurs in treating children with PKU with a special diet.

In autosomal recessive diseases, the affected person must have the same abnormal gene present on both chromosomes of a pair. This requires that the child receive the same abnormal gene from both parents (Figure 9-5). These parents, generally unaffected, are carrying the gene in a single dose and are called carriers. Carriers possessing one recessive gene generally have no manifestations of the disease, though in some cases of biochemical disorders, mild abnormalities can be detected in the carrier state.

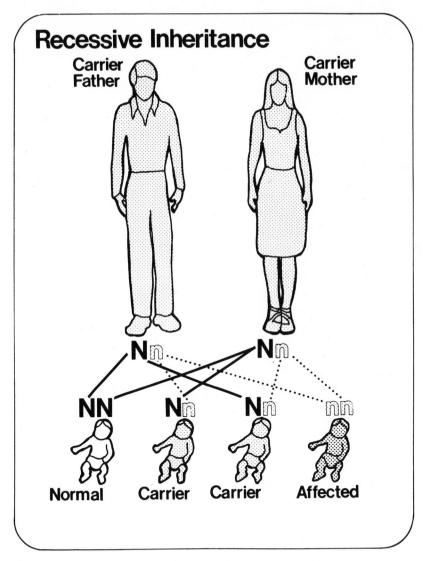

Figure 9-5   Recessive inheritance—*Both* parents, usually unaffected, carry a normal gene (N) which is generally sufficient for normal function despite the presence of its faulty counterpart (n). The odds in each pregnancy are: 1) a 25% risk of inheriting a "double dose" of n genes which may cause a serious birth defect, 2) a 25% chance of inheriting two Ns, thus being free of the faulty gene, and 3) a 50% chance of being a carrier like both parents. Adapted from: The New Human Genetics. DHEW Publ. No. (NIH) 76-662.

The disease will become manifest only when a carrier marries another individual carrying a similar defective gene. In any mating of this type, there is a 25% chance for the offspring to receive both abnormal genes and express the disease, a 50% chance for a child to have one abnormal gene and not express the disease but be a carrier, and a 25% chance for a completely normal child.

In a similar way, certain ethnic groups have increased rates of similar defective genes, and marriages between these groups show a higher incidence of recessive disease. This is seen in the Ashkenazi Jewish population which has a carrier trait for Tay-Sachs disease, which occurs in about one in every 30 people of this ethnic group. The black populations have a carrier rate for sickle cell anemia of about one in nine. Peoples from the Mediterranean area, the Italians and Greeks, have a high carrier type for thalassemia of approximately one in ten. The Norwegians have a high carrier frequency for phenylketonuria.

In the generation following parents who have a child manifesting a recessive disease, the likelihood of their normal, carrier children subsequently reproducing this disease is relatively small. This will vary with the amount of inbreeding occurring in the family and with the frequency of the abnormal gene in the mate's population. Because of the low frequency of similar genes occurring, the chances of producing a child with the disease become relatively small. In cases of specific disease entities, careful genetic counseling should be sought, as each case must be answered specifically.

Autosomal recessive disorders:

sickle cell anemia	infantile multicystic kidney
Tay-Sachs disease	disease
thalassemia	Wilson disease
cystic fibrosis	Werdnig-Hoffman disease
PKU	oculocutaneous albinism

X-linked, or sex-linked, recessive disorders have the same genetic considerations, only these genes are carried on the X chromosome. Because the male has only one X chromosome, and the Y chromosome does not exhibit any marked genetic influence, it is necessary for males to receive only one X chromosome containing a mutant gene to manifest the disease (Figure 9-6). In this type of disorder, the disease, then, is usually manifest in a male whose mother is a carrier. It is only in rare cases that the disease is manifest in a female, as she must have two abnormal genes received from both her parents. These conditions are quite rare and usually very severe.

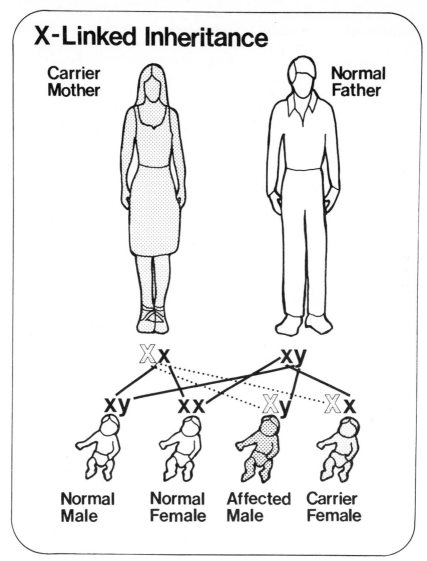

Figure 9-6 X-Linked inheritance—In the most common form, the female sex chromosomes of an unaffected mother carries one faulty gene (X) and one normal one (x). The father has normal male x and y chromosome complement. The odds for each *male* child are 50/50: 1) 50% risk of inheriting the faulty X and the disorder and 2) 50% chance of inheriting normal x and y chromosomes. For each *female* child, the odds are: 1) 50% risk of inheriting one faulty X, to be a carrier like mother and 2) 50% chance of inheriting no faulty gene. Adapted from: The New Human Genetics. DHEW Publ. No. (NIH) 76-662.

All male children of a carrier mother will have a 50% chance of having the disease. None of her daughters will exhibit the disease but will have a 50/50 chance of being a carrier.

If the affected male with an X-linked recessive disease has children, he can transmit this disease to none of his sons, as he only gives them the Y chromosome. All his daughters, however, will be carriers, as they receive one of their X chromosomes from the father. In the subsequent generation, 50% of the male children of these daughters will have the disease.

The problem of X-linked recessive disorders becomes complex when there is no family history of the disorder and it is not known whether the mother of the child is actually a carrier for this disease. In this situation, there is a possibility that the mutation could have occurred in the affected male, and therefore was not actually inherited. In some situations, there are straightforward biochemical or immunologic methods of identifying carriers. In other instances, there is no reliable carrier detection method. In these situations, careful genetic counseling is necessary and the empiric risks will vary with each individual case.

X-linked recessive disorders:

hemophilia	testicular feminization
Duchenne muscular	syndrome
dystrophy	X-linked ichthyosis
Fabry disease	glucose-6-phosphate
anhidrotic ectodermal	dehydrogenase
dysplasia	color blindness

Since 1950, there has been a rapidly expanding knowledge in the area of biochemical genetic disorders. These have generally been labeled as "inborn errors of metabolism." Basically, these are genetic errors occurring in the biochemical mechanism where there is an alteration in the production of certain specific enzymes. These enzymes control the rate and direction of chemical reactions within the body. Abnormal genes either result in the production of no enzyme or in the production of an abnormal enzyme which interferes with the normal pathways of metabolism. This then will result in the lack of production of necessary chemical substances or the accumulation of abnormal substances. Either of these two mechanisms can result in severe brain damage. Because these errors of metabolism are present at birth, the diseases become manifest early in life and damage to the central nervous system occurs early.

Many of these diseases are now treatable, usually by modifying the diet. Treatment must start extremely early in life—within the first few weeks—if severe brain damage is not to occur.

POLYGENIC DISORDERS

Polygenic disorders represent the cumulative effect of many genes that work in both a negative and positive way to produce disease. The influence of the environment and of such factors as nutrition, illness, physical and intellectual stimulation, play an important role in determining the ultimate degree of expression of these entities. Diabetes mellitus, hypertension, cleft palate, club foot, neural tube defects, and certain types of congenital heart disease are all some of our more common polygenic disorders. See Chapter 11 on medical syndromes for further information.

Frequent polygenic entities:

cleft palate	pyloric stenosis
club foot	nonspecific mental
neural tube defects	retardation
congenital heart disease	schizophrenia
diabetes mellitus	atopic allergic disease
hypertension	(hayfever, asthma)
hydrocephalus	Hirschsprung disease

It is not unusual to find that the parents of children with polygenic disease themselves appear normal. Because of the necessity for involving many genes in the development of these diseases, the frequency of subsequent children having the disorder is much less than that occurring in recessive and dominant mechanisms of transmission.

When a polygenic disease occurs in a child, there is, however, a definite increased risk of recurrence in subsequent children born to the same parents, over that of the general population. There is a baseline risk of 2% to 5% for recurrence in subsequent offspring providing there are no other close relatives having similar disability. If other members of the family are affected, the risk increases. Careful genetic counseling is necessary to determine the individual risks involved as they will vary with the number of affected members in the family. For this reason, individual counseling is necessary.

Neural tube defects (NTD), which occur in the United States in about one per 1000 births, appear to have a polygenic inheritance factor, as there is a risk of about 2% to 6% of having another child with NTD in subsequent offspring. The abnormalities occur in these children because of the failure of the neural tube in the embryo to form normally. In this early process of embryologic development, marked changes occur rapidly in the development of the nervous system. When the tube fails to fuse and develop properly, an abnormality occurs which can affect different areas of the nervous system. The type of abnormality depends on where and when the embryonic development failed. The child might be an encephalic, when there is a total failure of most of the brain to develop. Or he could have an encephalocele, with protrusion, usually through the back of the head, of an improperly developed brain. Meningomyeloceles are frequently manifested as a protrusion of the spinal cord at the lower end of the spine. The meningomyeloceles can be very mild causing no difficulties, or they can be extremely severe causing total paralysis of the lower extremities.

There is a considerable variation in the incidence of neural tube defects in different ethnic groups. There appears to be a high frequency in the Irish and a lower incidence in eastern Europeans. Geographic location appears also to play a possible role which might suggest some environmental factor causing the precipitation of difficulties. At present, it is impossible to establish any definite, consistent environmental agent which plays a role in causation. The disease can usually be diagnosed in utero (see the section on amniocentesis in Chapter 8) by finding an abnormally elevated level of alpha-feto-protein or by using ultrasound.

At present, the low incidence of the disease does not require the monitoring of all pregnancies for possible neural tube defects. Mothers having had one child with an NTD or a spontaneous abortion where the fetus showed evidence of neural tube abnormalities should have genetic counseling.

Club foot has an incidence of about one in 1500 to one in 1700 and is seen more often in males than in females. In cases of congenital club foot, a search for other causative factors such as chromosome abnormalities, abnormal uterine position, or congenital amniotic bands should be undertaken. Genetic counseling in individual cases is important.

Congenital hip dislocation has an incidence of about one in 1000 to one in 1200 births. A search for other causative factors should be undertaken before deciding that it is polygenic.

Congenital heart disease occurs in an estimated six to nine per 1000 births with defects varying from simple to complex. The defects may be nothing more than a simple defect in the septum of the heart which will cause no difficulties throughout the child's life and may even close. Or, there may be complex abnormalities that are incompatible with life.

These diseases might be diagnosable immediately after birth, or they might take several weeks or months before the condition becomes noticeable and before a heart murmur or other abnormality can be detected. Careful neonatal care and well-baby follow-up can detect most of these abnormalities very early in life.

Congenital heart disease is seen more frequently in certain types of genetic disease, particularly Down syndrome. It also is a frequent occurrence in teratogenic problems such as those caused by rubella or the phenylhydantoin syndrome.

Brothers and sisters of children having only a congenital heart disease (not part of another syndrome of congenital abnormalities) run a polygenic recurrence risk of 2% to 5%. Congenital heart disease affects both males and females equally, having no propensity for one sex over the other.

Familial mental retardation   One type of mental retardation, usually of mild to moderate severity, appears to "occur in families" and is relatively common. These people appear to be both chromosomally and biochemically normal. No specific or consistent abnormalities can be found throughout the family.

The offspring of couples with this mild form of retardation usually do not show any progressively increasing severity of retardation. There is some concern that perhaps these children suffer from a lack of stimulation in their early formative years, and this lack of stimulation tends to compound the problem. Early intervention programs are now being developed and provided for these children whenever they can be reached, diagnosed, and brought into a program. Headstart and preschool training are frequently very effective in developing the intellectual capacity of these children to their ultimate capability.

Schizophrenia, atopic allergies (eczemas, hayfever, etc), essential hypertension, and diabetes mellitus seem to fall into the polygenic classification. These diseases appear to cluster in families and to have a recognizable genetic risk of recurrence.

Though the risks in all polygenic traits are small, the previous occurrence of any of these disease entities in the family should alert parents to the possibility that the disease will recur. When indicated, careful physical and laboratory examinations should be undertaken for evaluation.

10 Mental Retardation

Mental retardation is a phenomenon occurring in a significant portion of the world's population. The causes are many and varied—in the majority of cases defying specific diagnosis or definition.

The official definition of mental retardation as published by the American Association of Mental Deficiency (AAMD) in the *Manual on Terminology and Classification in Mental Retardation* (see Appendix 3) is:

> Mental retardation refers to *sigificantly* subaverage, general intellectual functioning existing concurrently with deficits in adaptive behavior and manifested during the developmental period. Thus, subnormal intelligence is no longer the sole determinant of mental retardation, but the inability to adapt behaviorally to the world in which the person lives must exist concurrently as well.

It also involves a relationship of the person with his peers so that he is compared to the activities of normal people of his age and in his culture. Mental retardation denotes a level of behavioral performance without respect to etiology. It does not distinguish between the genetically inherited disorders, such as those associated with chromosomal or genetic abnormalities, and the retardation perhaps associated with psychosocial or cultural deprivation. Mental retardation is descriptive of the current behavior of the child and does not, by itself, imply a prognosis.

Adaptive behavior is defined as the effectiveness or the degree with which the individual meets the standards of personal independence and social responsibility expected of his age and cultural group. Since these expectations vary for different age groups, deficits of adaptive behavior will vary for different age groups, deficits of adaptive behavior will vary at different ages. Descriptions of adaptive behavior norms may be found in the *AAMD Manual* (see Appendix 4).

Intellectual functioning can be assessed by one or more of the standard intelligence quotient (IQ) tests. The two most frequently used tests are the Stanford-Binet and the Wechsler Intelligence Scale for Children. These intelligence tests require time and experience in administering, grading, and interpreting; proper interpretation of the scores requires a skilled and trained professional.

The AAMD has established levels of retardation—mild, moderate, severe, and profound which can be based upon IQ scores. A median or mean IQ of the population has been arbitrarily set at 100 which represents average intellectual functioning. A genius will have an IQ score of 135 to 170, and in some cases even higher. Retardation levels are shown in Table 10-1 below. It can be seen that there is a difference in scoring depending upon the type of test given, but essentially these tests will fall into the same scoring range.

Table 10-1
Retardation Levels

	IQ Range	
	Stanford-Binet	Wechsler
Mild	67–52	69–55
Moderate	51–36	54–40
Severe	35–20	39–25 (Extrapolated)
Profound	19 and below	24 and below (Extrapolated)

A child's IQ can be used as a general indication of potential capacity. It is important, however, that too much emphasis not be placed on a retarded child's IQ so that it masks the potential for improving his abilities if offered the proper educational training and environmental advantages.

If tests for IQ are not given accurately or if the person being tested either does not understand the directions or because of behavioral difficulties will not perform, the IQ scores on such a test might be totally erroneous. It should be emphasized that determination of mental retardation is dependent upon the finding of both a significantly low IQ and deficient adaptive behavior for the child's age and cultural setting.

Deficits in adaptive behavior will vary at different ages, and they may be reflected as follows: During infancy and early childhood, they will manifest in sensory-motor skills development; communication skills, including speech and language; self-help skills—dressing and toileting; and socialization—the ability to interact with other people. During childhood and early adolescence, defects in adaptive behavior may be reflected in poor application of basic academic skills to daily life activities, inability to use appropriate reasoning and judgment in the mastery of the environment; and the lack of social skills permitting participation in group activities and interpersonal relationships. During late adolescence and adult life, in addition to the above, deficits in vocational and social responsibilities and performances are also indicative of delayed adaptive behavior skills.

Normal patterns of child development are discussed in the first chapters of this book. It must be emphasized that these are broad guidelines. Minor or even major deviations may or may not be important. If, however, parents fear that development is delayed, it is important to seek professional care and evaluation. It should be sought early in the child's life, as early stimulation programs have proved effective in accelerating and developing the full potential of the child.

LEVELS OF RETARDATION

At the present time, the general descriptions used in designating mental retardation are mild, moderate, severe, and profound. See Table 10-1.

Mild mental retardation comprises approximately 75% of the total. Many of the mildly retarded are not recognized until they begin to fail academically in school, in kindergarten to the third grade. "Mildly retarded" is roughly equivalent to the educational term "educable." This child can usually learn simple academic skills, self-help skills, and can usually reach the scholastic equivalence of the fourth to fifth grades. Most of these children are educated in special education classes, and today many will complete this type of program through a high school curriculum. As adults, the majority of these people will disappear into the work force and many will marry. They will perform adequately socially and as employees as long as they are not required to engage in abstract thought or complex ideas.

Approximately 17% to 21% of the total group comprise the moderately retarded or the "trainable" group of people. These people usually will learn simple language and speech, perhaps some writing. Their self-help skills are delayed, but they are capable of learning the basic care needed to take care of themselves such as feeding, dressing, and toileting. Many can find jobs in sheltered workshops if they are available in the community. These people usually function fairly well in society with supervision. Institutionalization is usually not required.

The other 4% are the severely and profoundly retarded, the group having extremely low IQs and minimal adaptive behavior. These children's handicaps are frequently noticed at birth or shortly after; they show multiple difficulties including, in many cases, severe physical difficulties. A few of these severely retarded children will learn to walk, talk, and develop some self-help skills, but this may be minimal. Because of their extreme dependence and association of other chronic health conditions, many of these are institutionalized, either early in life or by adolescence. Many of these children die in infancy from complicating problems, either due to the primary disease causing their retardation, eg, Tay-Sachs disease, or because of secondary problems, eg, congenital heart disease.

What is the extent of the problem as it exists in the United States today? The overall retarded population is generally accepted to be 3%, comprising approximately 6 million Americans. Approximately 100,000 new cases are added each year. Approximately 4% of all children born are mentally retarded, falling below the general cutoff both in adaptive behavior and two standard deviations below the mean in IQ. Because these children are frequently severely damaged and affected with multiple handicaps, many of them will die early in life. In the adult population we find between 1% and 2% of the U.S. population are still classified as mentally retarded. Probably a significant percentage of this lost 2% adapt to their social environment and are lost to the collection of data.

The cost of supporting and maintaining the retarded population is enormous, being estimated as between $4.5 and $7 billion per year. The Department of Health, Education, and Welfare alone spent $1.7 billion in 1976 on programs for the retarded. Any child requiring institutionalization throughout his life can be expected to cost the taxpayers between $250,000 and $500,000. This in itself should be sufficient stimulation to develop programs to educate and train the retarded to their fullest capacity and make them capable of becoming active members of the work force rather than financial burdens to their family and to society.

Physiologic retardation, an inherited low IQ, may be a cause of many cases of mild to moderate retardation. Socioeconomic factors of poverty, lack of environmental stimulation, and differing cultural values can all be causative factors.

Parents should realize that unless their retarded child has significant other handicapping conditions, particularly serious heart disease, or is afflicted with one of the more serious progressive central nervous system diseases, the average life expectancy of a retarded child today is approaching 50 to 53 years.

CAUSES OF RETARDATION

Frequent questions asked of the professionals in developmental disabilities are, "What are the causes?" "What can we do about them?" "How can they be treated?" and "Can they be prevented in future children?"

Unfortunately, we are not adept at reaching a definitive diagnosis of the cause of retardation in every case. Even though 200 different specific causes of mental retardation have been identified, in 75% of the cases, a finite medical diagnosis cannot be assigned.

Many of these people in the "unknown" group are simply on the low end of the intelligence scale. Just as some people are tall and some are short, so are some people extremely intelligent, in the genius category, while others have an inherited low intelligence or a physiologic retardation.

Unfortunately, we cannot diagnose all the inborn errors of metabolism which probably occur. Certainly there are infections that are unknown and undiagnosed, and there is maldevelopment of the brain from causes we are incapable of understanding. Nor can we peer into the brain the way a repairman can look into the electronic circuit of a television, nor can we simply pull out and replace a circuit or worn tube or defective tuner. Perhaps someday not far in the future, electronic circuitry can be utilized to overcome certain brain damage or deficiencies. Work is already progressing in the fields of hearing and vision to perfect such electronic capabilities.

Mental retardation can be caused by certain infections and intoxications. These include, among others, congenital rubella or German measles, congenital syphilis, toxoplasmosis, and any viral or bacterial infection causing an encephalitis or meningitis. Intoxications due to toxemia of pregnancy, lead poisoning, or poisoning by other heavy metals, eg, mercury, hyperbilirubinemia, the jaundice occurring with Rh sensitization, can cause severe brain damage, called kernicterus.

Trauma caused by injury prenatally, mechanical injury at birth, absence of oxygen in utero or after birth, and postnatal injury can all cause significant brain damage.

Many metabolic diseases can cause abnormal central nervous system functioning. The majority of these are genetic diseases, and several will be discussed in greater detail later. These errors in metabolism include such malfunctions as the neuronal lipid storage diseases—such as Tay-Sachs—where there is an accumulation of abnormal fatty substances in the individual neurons in the brain.

Galactosemia, the glucogen storage diseases, and fructosemia are disorders in the carbohydrate or starch and sugar metabolism.

Among the amino acid disorders, phenylketonuria or PKU is probably the most common.

Some diseases involve abnormal metabolism of minerals. Wilson disease, caused by an abnormal metabolism of copper, is an example.

Endocrine or glandular disturbances are some of the more common causes of retardation. Congenital hypothyroidism, or cretinism, occurs in approximately 1 in 5000 live births.

Significant central nervous system damage can be caused by gross brain disease caused by infiltrative tumors, neurofibromatosis, or von Recklinghausen disease. Abnormal blood vessel development with blood vessel tumors and degenerative diseases occurring in the cerebral white matter can all cause significant to severe mental retardation.

Some diseases occurring later in life are degenerative in nature; the nerves form normally then degenerate. The most common among these is Huntington chorea, an autosomal dominant genetic disease, which manifests itself usually in midlife.

We have to classify some of our malformations and maldevelopments as due to unknown prenatal influence. These include the cerebral malformations such as anencephaly where there is a lack of formation of a major portion of the brain. Hydrocephaly, an accumulation of fluid within the ventricles in the brain, may or may not cause significant mental retardation, depending on the amount of damage to the cortex of the brain before therapy is instituted. Microcephaly, characterized by small heads from unknown causes, occurs because of a lack of sufficient central nervous system tissue; there is usually a marked decrease in intelligence.

Chromosomal abnormalities are some of the more readily identifiable types of diseases, accounting for 15% to 16% of the mentally retarded. The most common of these is Down syndrome in which there is a trisomy, or an extra No. 21 chromosome. Trisomy-13 and trisomy-18 are also rare but identifiable. Chromosomal abnormalities involving the X chromosome, such as Turner or Klinefelter syndromes, may or may not be associated with mental retardation. (See Chapter 9.)

Gestational disorders, particularly prematurity and postmaturity and, in more recent times, the fetal alcohol and smoking syndromes have been identified as causing potential damage to the central nervous system of the unborn child. These were discussed in Chapter 8.

DIAGNOSIS

How is the mentally retarded child diagnosed? The typical mentally retarded child, comprising approximately 75%, would be seen at the physician's office after being referred from the school as showing significantly delayed educational development and progressing more slowly than his peers.

Mild to moderate mental retardation can be caused by psychosocial disadvantages. This becomes apparent particularly in the crowded ghettos where there is little cultural or social stimulation, either in the home or the environment. A lack of early stimulation can be significant in creating an inability to develop to full intellectual capacity.

The more profound or seriously retarded usually will be noticed earlier. If a child has definite physical abnormalities, particularly abnormalities involving his face and head, he will usually be evaluated at a much earlier age. If the child fails to reach motor development milestones by being markedly delayed in sitting, walking, or talking, professional consultation is frequently obtained when the child is two to three years of age. A retarded child from a lower socioeconomic group or a unique culture may perform well within that culture and may not be identified until later in life if he is identified at all. This delay, unfortunately, compounds the difficulties in the development of intellectual capabilities.

A concerned parent might ask, "When should I seek help?" The best advice we can offer is that professional help should be sought at any time it is felt a child is not reaching the developmental milestones that were discussed earlier in this book. No one should be afraid to be a concerned parent and consult with professionals whenever there is reason to believe that there is some difficulty.

Perhaps the greatest mistake that can be made is to adopt a "let's wait and see" attitude. This might be permissible in certain circumstances if the child is not markedly delayed and particularly if he is not delayed in more than one sphere. The best advice still will remain: If in doubt, search us out.

In the process of a physical examination, careful attention should be given to vision and hearing. A child with serious visual defects, unable to see his environment with any clarity, may act retarded. If a child is totally blind, this usually will be recognized early in life and intervention programs can be started early.

Hearing loss can cause a child to appear to be retarded. There are many cases on record, particularly in years past, of children being placed in institutions for the retarded when their only problem was that of being deaf. These children usually appear very quiet and inattentive; they do not follow sounds, and speech may be defective or delayed. Fortunately, testing procedures are being done in many newborn nurseries and most well-baby clinics to evaluate, at least crudely, auditory capabilities.

The time of acquisition of speech is varied; arbitrarily most people dealing with mentally retarded children become concerned if the child is not speaking by age two, or at least saying short sentences of two to three words. However, if the child has normal physical findings, if his head circumference is normal, if his motor development has been normal to date, and if he is following verbal commands so that his auditory perception is good, he is probably not retarded. Some children who are not mentally retarded develop speech late and do not speak single words until approximately 18 months and do not develop effective language until three years. If there is concern, evaluation by a speech therapist might be indicated.

In many cases, dermatoglyphics—looking at finger-, hand-, and foot-prints—are helpful in establishing a diagnosis, as characteristic patterns are seen in certain syndromes.

In searching for congenital abnormalities, the physician, or for that matter even the parent, should take careful measurement of the circumference of the head at its widest point. This measurement, called the OFC, or occipital-frontal circumference, will indicate if there is an unusually large or small head. Small or large heads both can be associated with mental retardation. Both of these conditions, however, can also be seen in normal people and can be part of an inherited constitution.

Abnormal reflexes or a poor muscle tone (so that the child appears "floppy") may indicate central nervous system damage. Poor suckling or swallowing or severe feeding difficulties early in neonatal life might require evaluation by a health professional.

Convulsions in the newborn should be evaluated very carefully as to cause. Hypoglycemia, low blood sugar, or hypocalcemia, low blood calcium, can both cause neonatal convulsions. If untreated, these can cause severe and irreversible brain damage. Convulsions occurring later in life of the child should be evaluated by a health professional as to cause and therapy started if indicated.

Emotional disorders can cause children to appear to be retarded. Chronic anxieties and frank depression can cause school failure and poor performance on intelligence tests. This type of functional retardation can usually be alleviated with careful counseling and educational programs.

Autism and childhood schizophrenia, which are primary emotional disturbances can be misdiagnosed as mental retardation. These are discussed more fully in Chapter 16, on emotional disorders.

Children with perceptual abnormalities may present with academic skill difficulties and may be mislabeled as mildly retarded. Poor memory and disturbances in eye-hand coordination, visual, or auditory perception may be involved. These children can be differentiated by careful psychologic testing.

Children with cerebral palsy may or may not be mentally retarded depending on the extent of the brain damage. Cerebral palsy is discussed in Chapter 13. Certain chronic diseases, particularly kidney and heart disorders can cause a child to develop a small stature and appear to be retarded. Proper testing can diagnose these children, and with proper treatment of their primary disease, their physical features will usually return more to normal.

LABORATORY TESTS

In most states today, a screening examination during the newborn period is mandatory for phenylketonuria (PKU); sometimes for other diseases as well. PKU occurs in approximately one in 11,000 live births throughout the United States. If found very early in life, treatment by the modification of diet is possible. Perhaps more important and increasingly used today is the early newborn evaluation of thyroid function searching for congenital hypothyroidism, or cretinism. This occurs in one in 5000 live births, and again must be treated very early to prevent permanent brain damage.

In evaluating a child who appears to be delayed, laboratory work should include a screen for the known inborn errors of metabolism, looking for amino acid abnormalities. Where indicated, studies of abnormal sugar and fat metabolism should also be investigated.

Some 20 to 30 different conditions can be diagnosed by laboratory tests early in life. These include many of the inborn errors of metabolism such as PKU, galactosemia, homocystinuria, maple syrup urine disease, histidinemia, methyl-malonic aciduria, as well as hypothyroidism. In many of these cases, mental retardation may be prevented or ameliorated if diet or other medical therapy is imposed early in life.

Parents should be advised that in screening programs of this type for many diseases, if a positive report is received, further laboratory testing must be done to arrive at a specific, firm diagnosis. Screening tests tend to be very sensitive and occasional false positive reports occur. Follow-up laboratory testing is mandatory to arrive at a specific and definitive diagnosis. Follow-ups should be done immediately upon receipt of a positive screening test as time is extremely important.

Other laboratory tests may or may not be necessary. If indicated, a complete blood count, urinalysis, TORCH* screen and tuberculosis skin test will give a general screening for many potential diseases. X-rays might be indicated in certain types of problems and might include x-rays of the skull to see if there are any obvious brain growth abnormalities. X-rays might be taken of the kidneys, chest, or long bones in certain specific cases when looking for diseases of the kidneys or when there is a question of dwarfism. Normal bone x-rays will usually rule out any heavy metal poisoning as changes in the x-ray findings can be diagnostic.

Cytogenetic studies, looking at chromosomes, is extremely important when any genetic abnormality is suggested. This is discussed more fully in Chapter 9. Certainly chromosome studies are indicated in any child that at birth looks as if he might have Down syndrome. There are children born with other multiple anomalies which may or may not fit a known syndrome; the study of chromosomes in these children may help to reach a specific diagnosis.

Electroencephalograms, EEGs, may or may not be of some value. Most neurologists do not believe that they should be done in all cases of mental retardation, though all will agree that brain wave tracings should be done in any children suspected of having a seizure disorder.

Because of the increased incidence of abnormal brain patterns in mentally retarded people, there is a high frequency of abnormal EEGs. In most cases, EEGs are not diagnostic for specific types of mental retardation. They will diagnose specific types of seizure disorders, and they are capable of pinpointing areas of the brain with abnormal or absent electrical brain-wave patterns.

---

*TORCH—toxoplasmosis, rubella, cytomegalic inclusion disease, and herpes.

The CAT (computerized axial tomography) scan is becoming more and more useful in determining abnormalities of the brain. They are particularly useful in diagnosing tumors, cysts, abcesses, or any other abnormal growths within the skull. The CAT scan can be costly; charges range from $100 to $300.

Perhaps the most important thing in establishing or not establishing a diagnosis in a mentally retarded child is the conveying of this information to the parents. It is important that the physician or health professional discuss his findings with the parent in as great detail as possible. It is equally important that the parent search out this information and find answers to all his questions.

When approaching a physician with concerns, parents must be *specific* in delineating all their worries. An ideal method is to write these down in as great detail as possible so that each of the concerns will be discussed with the physician.

It is important to discuss emotional concerns, to share thoughts with the physician, and to give him insight into attitudes, frustrations, and possible guilt feelings concerning the child's retardation problems.

We find on many occasions that trivia become magnified to the point of causing real concerns. We have seen concerns regarding excessive smoking, drinking, or eating the wrong foods. One woman was concerned because she ate too much watermelon; her grandmother told her that the watermelon was probably what caused her child to be retarded. This is a totally erroneous concept, and it sounds silly, but it really happened. These concerns, even though they seem trivial, if they are important to the parent should be discussed with the physician.

Perhaps the most common mistake made by most physicians and parents is their difficulty in accepting borderline delays in development. Too often, physicians have been guilty of adopting a "wait and see" attitude. In the majority of cases where a child does not appear to be developing adequately by age two, careful evaluation by people working in the field of developmental disabilities should be considered. In any event, there is no harm in starting motor and sensory stimulation programs even on a normal child. If *any* doubt exists, stimulation programs should be begun and the child's development watched very carefully.

When there is evidence of definite delay, wherever possible the child should be referred to a multidisciplinary group that specializes in developmental disabilities. Groups of this type are being developed throughout the United States and are usually affiliated with either a university or a regional or community center. In the addenda to this book is a list of resource centers and agencies which can be helpful in securing proper diagnosis and treatment programs. If such a center is not available, a pediatrician interested in developmental disabilities or a pediatric neurologist can serve as a primary source of diagnosis and treatment.

Establishment of a definite diagnosis and prognosis is extremely difficult in these children. Because of the many variables affecting the child's potential, the ultimate prognosis in many cases can be nothing more than a guess. The child's response to his environment, stimulation, and his educational programs is completely variable. The ultimate capability of any one child in adulthood cannot be forecast with a great degree of accuracy.

TEACHING RETARDED CHILDREN

How can a retarded child be taught and trained?

By definition, intelligence includes the notion of the ability to learn. Since retarded children are less intelligent than average, they have a harder time learning than most people. However, they can learn; it just takes more time, more repetition, special techniques, and teaching geared to their particular needs and to their level of understanding.

Perhaps the biggest obstacles in the way retarded children learn are the expectations on the part of their parents and teachers. On the one hand, there is the expectation that if the child is retarded, he will not learn. On the other hand, there are unrealistic expectations of parents unwilling to accept that their child is retarded and that his learning process will be delayed.

In some respects, people have a strange habit of doing just what is expected of them. If they are expected to be smart, to learn, and to succeed, they will be successful. If, however, they are expected to be dumb and become failures, that is exactly what they will become. Retarded children can become failure-oriented, if that is what is expected of them. One of the most productive things that parents of retarded children can do is to know that their children can learn and to expect that with proper teaching they will learn. By focusing efforts on improving areas of strength still further, a great service is done to the child's self-concept.

The major aspect of teaching that needs adjustment for a retarded child is content—what is taught. Training in basic self-help, social, and economic skills are far more important for a retarded person than academic learning. For example, it is more important that a retarded boy be able to read words such as "Men's Room" and "Exit" than to be able to read "See Dick run." As a general rule of thumb, parents and teachers must remember that the practical, everyday skills which most of us take for granted are things which must be explicitly taught and retaught to retarded children.

Tasks must be presented to retarded children in small steps. Almost any action human beings engage in can be broken into a series of smaller actions. For example, eating a bit of mashed potatoes involves sitting at the table properly, picking up and holding a fork, scooping a bit of food off the plate, bringing the food to the mouth, opening the mouth, inserting the food, closing the mouth, and pulling the fork out of the mouth, then chewing and swallowing the food. In teaching a retarded child, it is often necessary to teach one step at a time.

The process of breaking a task down into its component parts is called "task analysis." Special education teachers in the community are a good resource to help parents analyze the tasks they wish to teach a retarded child. In addition, commercial packages are available providing task analyses of skills commonly taught to children. For example, a series of such packages, called CAMS (Curriculum and Monitoring Systems) programs, have been developed at the Utah State University Exceptional Child Center.

If one wishes to try task analysis, the first step is to write out all the steps one can think of to tasks to be taught. Then another family member or a friend should sit down and play the part of someone who knows how to do nothing except follow directions literally. The steps are read to him one by one, to see if what he does resembles the particular skill. If not, steps are adjusted accordingly.

Once a task is analyzed into its component parts, there is the problem of how to teach each step to the child. The first step should be demonstrated to the child; next, he should be guided through the step while saying what he is doing. This is continued giving a little less assistance each time, until the child is performing the step on his own. Each successful attempt should be followed immediately by a reward (more about this later). When the child has mastered the first step, the second step is taught in the same manner. Then steps one and two are chained together. The third step is taught and added to the first two steps. Continuing in this fashion, the child performs the entire act.

Sometimes, a retarded child will get "stuck" at one point in learning a task. That is, he will just not be able to get the hang of the step being taught. When this happens, it is necessary to bridge the gap between the last step he mastered and the step he is stuck on, by making up a new step which is halfway between the two steps. For example, if a child just cannot seem to learn to bring a spoon from his plate to his mouth, an intermediate step can be created by positioning his hand halfway to his mouth and teaching him to bring it the rest of the way up.

We live in an achievement-oriented society. Most of us are motivated to take care of ourselves and to learn new things. However, retarded children may not have these motivations. In order for them to be willing to put forth the effort to learn, we must make it worth their while by providing artificial motivation. To motivate a child, it is necessary to select some sort of small reward that is easy to administer, that the child understands, and that you know is rewarding to the child. Spinach would not be a good reward if the child does not like spinach. Points that can be earned and later traded in for something are not good rewards for a child with a mental age of under seven years who cannot really grasp the concept of numbers. Small bits of candy or raisins or other food are usually good rewards, provided that the child likes the kind of food being offered.

When a good reward has been found, it should be given to the child *immediately* after he successfully performs the task or step that he is being taught. At the same time he is rewarded, he might be told "Good job," "Great!," "I like the way you're trying," or "Very good." The variations are endless. Eventually, the child will be willing to work for the praise, and the candy can be cut down to every second, fifth, or even tenth success.

No child will be everything exactly right every time; there will be failures. It is very important that the child not be punished, criticized, or belittled for failing. The best approach is not to give the reward and to say something like "Not quite—let's try again," and try the task another time.

Children have short attention spans, and this is especially true of retarded children. If one exceeds a child's attention span by trying to drill something into him for hours on end, he will begin to find the task quite aversive. So, when teaching a retarded child, it is best to keep the teaching sessions short. Three ten-minute sessions are better than one thirty-minute session.

Retarded children have difficulty remembering things for short periods of time. However, with repeated drill and practice, their long-term memory is adequate. So, in order to teach a retarded child effectively, one must be patient, persistent, repetitious, and consistent. Short-term, intensive teaching efforts will be largely unsuccessful. Rather, retarded children learn best and retain what they learn longest when teaching begins early in their lives and continues as a steady repetitious life-long process.

We recently heard from the mother of a 37-year-old man with Down syndrome. Even to this day, this mother is working with this man to help him increase his speaking and writing vocabulary. He has devised his own form of dictionary, keeps the words on a cork board in his room, and becomes extremely excited when he learns a new word and learns how to use it over and over again.

As with all children, teaching retarded children is not entirely a matter of teaching them new skills. The learning process also involves the elimination of undesirable behaviors, such as temper tantrums. Retarded children tend, more than brighter children, to engage in repetitious and self-destructive behaviors, such as rocking and head-banging. If the undersirable behaviors are dangerous or extremely noxious, it may be necessary to suppress them by punishing the child. However, psychologists generally do not like the use of punishment, because it can have many undesirable side effects. So, usually the best way to eliminate an undesirable behavior is with a "time out" procedure as the form of punishment.

To use a time-out procedure with a child, one selects a small, secluded area of the house such as a small room, a large unused closet, or a bare corner of a room screened off from the rest of the room. This area is kept free from all toys, diversions, pictures, people, or anything else that the child might find rewarding. When he engages in an undesirable behavior such as a temper tantrum, he is taken with a minimum of fuss to the time-out area. In as few words as possible, he is told why he is being taken there (that is, what the behavior is which is not allowed). Then he is left in the time-out area for approximately five minutes without interacting with him during this time. Time outs should be brief; they are merely short pauses from normal activity, not punishments or solitary confinements. They should never end while the child is in the midst of a tantrum; he must calm down before he is allowed to resume his normal activities.

This procedure might be recognized as a variation of the old "go to your room" punishment. The difference is that rooms can be cozy places with lots of playthings, while time-out areas are places where there is basically nothing to do. If time out is properly implemented, the child will eventually learn that misbehavior results in being taken away from the opportunity to do anything rewarding and that it is a lot more fun to not misbehave.

Toilet training is a type of learning which is often particularly important to parents of retarded children, for a toilet-trained child is certainly more pleasant to have around the house than one who is not. Profoundly retarded, institutionalized individuals may require special toilet training methods which utilize gimmicks such as moisture-sensitive, buzzer-equipped underpants. For most retarded children, however, toilet training can be accomplished in the same manner as for normal children, as outlined in Chapter 6, on self-help development. With retarded children, the process must be made more explicit, and it takes more time and effort. Like all other development milestones, toilet training is usually delayed and should not be attempted until the child is ready. The age of the child should have no bearing upon the time of instigation of training; some will train at two years of age, some not until ten.

A record of the time of the child's bowel movements can be kept until it is possible to predict their occurrence fairly accurately. Training can begin by taking the child to the potty shortly before a bowel movement is expected. Successes are rewarded lavishly. Working backward from this point, the child is taught to lower his own pants, to walk to the bathroom unassisted when asked to, to indicate (with a single word) the need to use the bathroom, and finally to perform the entire process himself. Once the child is able to indicate the need to go to the bathroom, accidents should be treated by having the child assist, to the degree that he is capable, in cleaning himself up. When bowel training is accomplished, bladder training can proceed in the same manner.

If more detail than this regarding toilet training is desired, or if there are problems in toilet training a child, a child psychologist in the community will be able to design an individualized toilet training program. In addition, commercially published, formally structured toilet training programs are available. Again, an example of such a program is the Utah State University Exceptional Child Center's CAMS Self-Help Program.

A retarded child places considerable demands upon a family. Teaching and raising a retarded child requires patience and persistence. However, if viewed as human beings with human emotional needs and as children who can learn and who will learn if given the proper opportunity, the majority of retarded children can become useful, productive, and at least partially self-sufficient adults.

11 Medical Syndromes

In this chapter we will discuss briefly some of the more common medical syndromes. The interested reader is referred to suggested readings in Appendix 3 for further information on these and other syndromes.

ABNORMAL CHROMOSOME NUMBER

Trisomy-13 or Patau Syndrome

This syndrome is caused by an extra No. 13 chromosome. The etiology, as in all trisomies, has not been firmly established, though it tends to occur in older mothers. The incidence of trisomy-13 is about one in 5000 births.

The clinical features include a variety of developmental and physical defects. All the infants are retarded, extremely jittery as infants, have difficulty breathing, and frequently appear to be deaf. Epilepsy is present in two-thirds of these children.

The head size is usually small, frequently with small eyes. A harelip and a cleft palate are present in the vast majority of cases. Other defects of the ears and eyes are also frequent. It is not unusual for these infants to have extra fingers and toes with frequent flexion deformities of the hands. These children usually die prior to one year of age. Diagnosis is confirmed by chromosome studies that show an extra No. 13 chromosome.

At present, there is no specific treatment for these children, although surgical repair of defects and symptomatic therapy may be undertaken.

Trisomy-18 or Edward Syndrome

Trisomy-18 occurs in approximately one in 6500 births. The mothers are usually in the older age group with an average age of 32 to 34 years. The etiology is unknown but is probably due to a failure of the chromosomes to separate during the development of the eggs or sperm.

These infants fail to thrive; showing poor growth and eating habits, with early evidence of developmental retardation. They usually have small heads and jaws with low-set and malformed ears. Flexion deformities of the joints are quite common, and the children have abnormal-looking feet with a curved heel called "rocker-bottom feet."

Death usually occurs in these children in infancy prior to 18 months of age. However, there are cases recorded where some of these children lived to be considerably older. The authors have recently seen a case of trisomy-18 in an eight-year-old girl. Her parents, unfortunately, had been advised that she would undoubtedly die within a year or year and a half and to do nothing but take her home and "love her." When seen, this child had severe contraction deformities of her legs, and no attempt had been made at any intervention program for her. It is our feeling that stimulation programs should be carried out on all these children within the limits of their capacities.

Cri du Chat Syndrome

Cri du chat or cat-cry syndrome is accompanied by severe mental retardation, a characteristic facial appearance, and abnormal skin changes. This disorder is named after the infant's cry in the nursery which sounds like the mewing of a cat.

In these cases, chromosomal aberrations have been found with a small piece of chromosome material missing from the short arm of chromosome 5 (Figure 11-1).

These children are severely retarded, have small heads, and a severe failure to thrive. Several of these children have lived to several years of age; early intervention programs are indicated.

Trisomy-21 or Down syndrome is discussed in Chapter 12. There are many other syndromes associated with minor abnormalities of the chromosomes. Almost all of them result in severe changes in the physical characteristics of the child, and most are associated with mild to severe retardation. These changes in the autosomes used to represent a small addition or deletion and can occur in most of the chromosomes Nos. 1 to 22. Each of these must be diagnosed individually and will present as rather characteristic syndromes. These are discussed in great length in Jean De Grouchy's book, *Clinical Atlas of Human Chromosomes*.

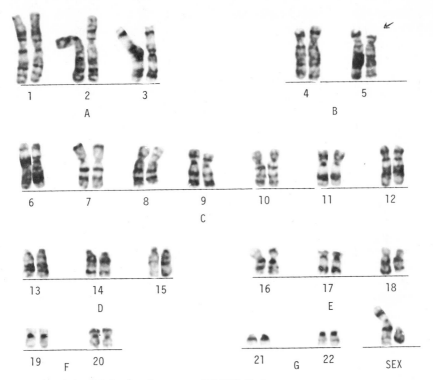

Figure 11-1   Cri du chat karyotype (46 XY, 5p-).

SEX CHROMOSOME ABNORMALITIES

All sex chromosome syndromes involve abnormalities of either the X or the Y chromosome, or both. In the majority of these difficulties there is either an extra chromosome or a missing chromosome.

Nondisjunction, or failure to separate during formation of the sex cells, is probably the basis for all abnormalities in the sex chromosomes. The two X chromosomes in the female or the XY chromosome in the male normally divide into single chrmosomes in the gametes. Mosaicism may result when nondisjunction takes place after conception, when the embryo is forming. This was discussed in Chapter 9, "Genetics."

An apparently normal child may have aberrations of the sex chromosomes as many children with an absent X chromosome or one more than normal are only diagnosed after they reach pubescence.

Turner Syndrome

Turner syndrome is an abnormality of the sex chromosome number accompanied by certain physical and endocrinologic features. In these children there is an absence of one of the X chromosomes in a phenotypically female child. These children will have a chromosomal count of 45, XO, with an absent or missing X chromosome (Figure 11-2).

The incidence of Turner syndrome is estimated at about one in 3000 live births; we frequently find evidence of karyotypes, 45, XO, in material obtained from a spontaneous abortion.

A person with Turner syndrome can usually be diagnosed early in life. The physical stature is rather short and stocky with the linear growth pattern delayed. These children usually have a wide chest with broadly spaced nipples, and a skin fold or webbing of the neck. Ears are sometimes low-set, and there is often a low back hairline. At puberty these children fail to mature, and usually do not develop secondary sex characteristics, lacking normal breast development or axillary and pubic hair. They have hormonal imbalances apparently due to failure of development of the ovaries.

Treatment to date is based on hormone replacement therapy and surgical repair of associated defects. In most patients, the hormone therapy produces breast development with pigmentation surrounding the nipple, uterine growth, and young girls, when treated with cyclic hormone

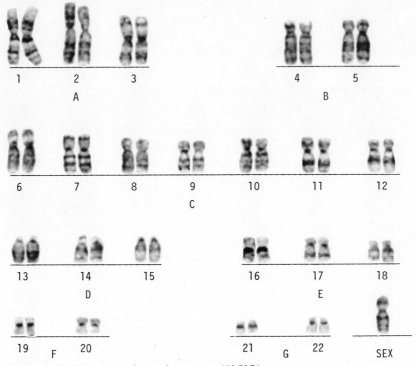

Figure 11-2 Turner syndrome karyotype (45 XO).

therapy, will have menstrual periods. These individuals, however, remain sterile because their ovaries are usually not developed and they do not produce eggs. There are occasional cases, usually in people with a mosaic Turner syndrome, where there have been pregnancies, but these are rare, and the incidence of chromosome abnormalities in the offspring is high.

Klinefelter Syndrome

This is a syndrome found in young males, though it may not be diagnosed until puberty when there is a primary failure of development of the male genitals. These people are frequently tall, asthenic, and have extremely small testicles that do not produce sperm. Male hormones are produced, however, so that secondary sex characteristics develop in these young men. Several cases referred to the author have presented as part of a sterility workup after these patients had been married for a period of time.

The chromosomal abnormality in Klinefelter syndrome is the presence of an extra X chromosome in a phenotypic male. This complement of XXY is most common, though other complements of XXXY or XXXXY have been reported (Figure 11-3).

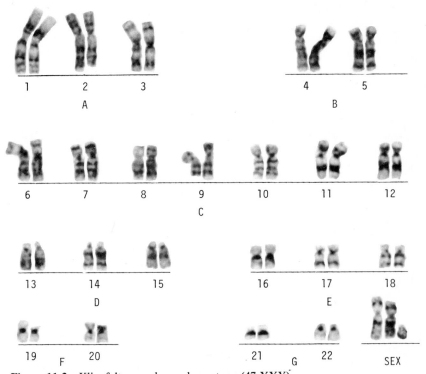

Figure 11-3 Klinefelter syndrome karyotype (47 XXY).

Generally, mental retardation is not present, but with cases of three- or four-X Klinefelter, retardation might be a problem.

Treatment of boys with Klinefelter syndrome is a testosterone replacement therapy in those with subnormal levels. There still is, however, an absence of sperm production, and these individuals remain sterile.

Hermaphroditism

A hermaphrodite or a pseudohermaphrodite is an individual having a discrepancy between the gonadal structures (testes or ovaries) and the external genitalia. A true hermaphrodite possesses both ovarian and testicular tissue. Children with this disorder have a normal complement of sex chromosomes. The cause of this entity is unknown.

A diagnosis can be made only when a biopsy demonstrates that both male and female gonadal tissues are present in the same person.

Most of these individuals have an XX chromosome complement, and as yet there is no adequate explanation as to why there is testicular tissue in patients lacking a Y, or male chromosome.

These children with intersex abnormalities should be treated. The general phenotype and the sex they assumed during rearing are more important than actual chromosome studies in determining which sex will be assigned the individual. Ideally, the sex of rearing should be established during infancy. Most medical authorities agree that surgical intervention may be helpful and agree that the sex of rearing should be changed only in cases of very young infants. For this reason it is imperative that the diagnosis be confirmed as early as possible so that a sex decision can be made. It is important to avoid possible endocrine imbalance and the psychological problem which may accompany any abnormal or faulty development at puberty.

AUTOSOMAL RECESSIVE SYNDROMES

Inborn errors of metabolism are usually biochemical genetic disorders which interfere with normal metabolism in the body. These genetic problems create errors in the body's chemical reactions, which are vital to produce energy and maintain normal cellular function. These errors might involve only certain types of cells in the body, eg, nerve cells, or they might be widespread, involving the metabolism of many of the body's organ systems.

A perhaps oversimplified explanation is that the basic mechanism causing the development of disease is usually the lack of an enzyme necessary to a biochemical reaction in the body. Or an enzyme may be produced which interferes with normal biochemical reactions. The genes in the body control, at the cellular level, the formation of specific enzymes. There are many hundreds of these enzymes, and their production is dependent upon a specific gene which is present on one of the 46 chromosomes. The enzymes are necessary to control the rate and direction of chemical reactions within the body. Sometimes several enzymes are required and may be coupled with coenzyme factors to accomplish these chemical changes. If a mutant or abnormal gene appears in the cell, a proper enzyme is not manufactured and the correct biochemical reaction does not take place. As a result of this, there may be an accumulation of abnormal substances or a failure to produce substances vital and necessary to the basic metabolism of the cell.

Most of these gene mutations causing inborn errors of metabolism are inherited in an autosomal recessive fashion. Most of these diseases appear early in life, and damage to the central nervous system will occur early because of the rapid accumulation of abnormal metabolic products or the damaging absence of critical chemical substances. There are many types of inborn errors of metabolism not associated with mental retardation or other physical handicaps. For these the interested reader is referred to suggested readings in the appendix to this book.

The inborn errors of metabolism can involve disorders of protein, carbohydrate, or lipid metabolism; in addition, a specific group is involved with connective tissue disorders. It should be reemphasized that these involve, with few exceptions, enzyme defects and may involve many different organs or cell systems.

Disorders of Amino Acid Metabolism

Phenylketonuria or PKU   This is the most commonly known of the aminoacidurias. In this disease, the body is unable to produce a specific enzyme needed to metabolize the amino acid phenylalanine to tyrosine. There is a lack, or reduced supply, of phenylalanine hydroxylase in children born with this disease. It is now believed that other enzymes may be involved in this complex metabolic disorder.

Historically, PKU is extremely interesting as it was the first inborn error of metabolism shown definitely to cause mental retardation. It was also the first of the inborn errors of metabolism that responded to therapy by diet modification.

The incidence of PKU in the United States today is about one in 10,000 to 11,000 live births. PKU appears to be more common among individuals of northern European stock and least common among blacks. It is estimated that about one in 50 to 100 people of Caucasian stock are carriers for PKU.

Children with PKU not diagnosed in early infancy and untreated show an early impairment of intelligence which becomes more marked with age and leads to severe to profound retardation in adulthood. These children are frequently light-haired and blue-eyed due to the under-production of tyrosine which is necessary to produce pigment in skin and eyes. Seizures are frequent, being found in 25% to 40% of the patients. Other symptoms suggestive of motor defects often associated with cerebral palsy are frequent.

A definite diagnosis requires laboratory analysis of the urine, blood, or both. The test used in most laboratories today, and used in mass screening programs, is a determination of the phenylalanine level in the blood. In the event elevated levels of phenylalanine are found on a screening test, a second test is done to determine the actual presence or absence of phenylketonuria.

The levels of phenylalanine in newborn screening programs have been set purposely low to avoid missing any potential disease. Ideally, an infant should have received some feedings of milk (the best source for phenylalanine) for at least 48 hours prior to the time he is screened for PKU. This is not always accomplished because mothers leave the hospital and go home earlier than in previous years, sometimes before the 48-hour period. It is felt that the low levels ascertained in screening procedures will still pick up the children with the disease.

Some mild variants found in the screening programs may not be due to a primary defect in phenylalanine metabolism. These require more definitive chemical determinations, which are available in most good laboratories.

Treatment is specific, requiring a diet low in, although not entirely devoid of, substances containing phenylalanine, which occur naturally in many foods. This requires a high intake of certain synthetic foods, especially synthetic milks that are specially formulated for children with PKU.

Treatment is usually quite successful if begun early in life, within weeks of birth. When started this early, extensive brain damage usually does not occur, and the children will grow up almost normally. IQs may be slightly depressed when compared to those of brothers and sisters not having PKU, but they usually do not fall into the mentally retarded range.

The time requirement for continuing the diet is still a matter of some concern. It appears, in many cases, that it may be discontinued in middle childhood, probably because brain development is usually almost complete by age three to four. It is also possible that metabolic pathways are developed preventing further damage to the nerve cells in the central nervous system.

A new problem now arising is that some of the children treated for PKU are now young adults and in the childbearing years. Women with PKU treated in early childhood and now off their severely restricted diets have elevated levels of phenylalanine in their blood. These excessive levels can be transmitted across the placenta, and an embryo and fetus can be severely damaged prior to birth. Recommendations at this time to women with PKU are that they return to their restrictive diets at least several months before conceiving and that they continue these diets throughout pregnancy. Women who have done this appear to deliver normal children without evidence of intrauterine brain damage. Long-term follow-up studies are still in progress.

Maple syrup urine disease is a severe, fatal inherited disease involving an abnormality in the metabolism of certain amino acids. The amino acids leusine, isoleusine, and valine accumulate in the body, eventually overflowing into the urine and giving the urine a characteristic maple syrup odor. This is a very rare disease with an incidence of about one in 300,000 live births.

The symptoms occurring in the first week of life consist of convulsions, difficulties in feeding, failure to thrive, and breathing difficulties. Most children die within the first years of life. Vomiting is frequent, and the children are all severely mentally retarded.

This disease can be demonstrated by the excessive amounts of these three amino acids in the blood and urine.

Attempts at treatment in recent years have included a variation in diet with strict dietary controls. Some improvement has been reported, but the disease is so rare that long-term trials have not been accomplished to date.

Homocystinuria is an inborn error of metabolism caused by an absence of the enzyme cystathionine synthetase. It is inherited as an autosomal recessive disease. These children present with early mental retardation, large livers, and are frequently found to have flushed cheeks; they may develop skeletal abnormalities caused by a low calcium content in their bones. Cataracts and dislocations of the lenses of the eyes are frequent. This disease, which occurs in about one in 10,000 to 15,000 live births, is treated by a diet controlling the intake of the amino acids methionine and cystine, with supplementation by massive doses of pyridoxine and some folic acid.

There are at least 30 to 40 other anomalies in amino acid metabolism with an incidence reported of one in 25,000 to 500,000 live births. Readers interested in further information are referred to suggested readings in Appendix 3 on metabolic errors and birth defects.

The classic view on these inborn errors of metabolism suggests that there is only one enzyme involved, resulting from a single gene mutation. The basic concept still remains valid, but new information suggests that perhaps there are several, if not many, genes involved in the metabolic abnormalities. As a result, deficiency of an enzyme may be due to more than one abnormal gene. This will account for some of the laboratory variations seen in studies of these diseases. There may be modification of the genetic systems that in turn modify and regulate the development and destruction of the metabolities. This is a very complex biochemical problem.

Carbohydrate Metabolism Diseases

The sugars and starches used by the body have a complex though orderly metabolism. Disorders of carbohydrate metabolism occur when genetic abnormalities prevent the production of necessary enzymes. Where these enzymes are deficient, there is a build-up of substances in the blood and in the urine. Most of these diseases are inherited as autosomal recessives. Common to all of them are failure to thrive, vomiting, low blood sugars, retarded growth, and findings of excessive quantities of carbohydrates or abnormal carbohydrates in the blood and urine. Most of the diseases are treatable by dietary restriction if diagnosed early in life.

Galactosemia is a rare inborn error of metabolism with a reported incidence varying from one in 40,000 to one in 187,000 live births. The child is noted to have an enlarged liver, does not grow and develop correctly, and exhibits a failure to thrive.

Galactosemia appears to be due to a deficiency in the enzyme galactose-1-phosphouridyl transferase, which converts galactose to glucose in the body. This results in damage to individual cells and to organs through an accumulation of galactose. Beside the failure to thrive and general listlessness, there is a noticeable enlargement of the liver and spleen accompanied by vomiting, diarrhea, and cataracts. Convulsions are frequent due to a fluctuating low blood sugar. Mental retardation is a consequent result of the general failure to thrive. In these children, the ingestion of large quantities of galactose can lead to convulsions and to brain damage.

Treatment consists of the institution of a galactose-free diet. As galactose is the major sugar found in milk, all milk and milk products must be omitted from this diet. Commercially produced substitutes are available and can provide adequate nutrition to an infant. The diet can gradually be modified as the child matures, permitting the ingestion of more and more foods as long as the galactose is kept to a minimum.

Screening for galactosemia is being instituted in more states throughout the country, as it is a treatable disease. If not carefully treated early in life, it causes severe retardation.

Fructosuria is an extremely rare autosomal recessive disease involving a metabolic block in the utilization of the sugar fructose. It is estimated that fructosuria occurs in about one in every 100,000 to 200,000 live births.

A deficiency of the liver enzyme aldolase interferes with the initial metabolic step in the metabolism of fructose. This results in an increased level of lactic acid in the blood and a rise in the blood and urine levels of fructose. The main clinical symptoms of fructosuria are similar to those of galactosuria except that no cataracts occur in fructosuria. Also a low magnesium level accompanies fructosuria with a resultant increase in central nervous system excitability. Treatment consists of elimination of fructose from the diet with the addition of high doses of folic acid in some cases.

Hereditary fructose intolerance is a benign form of fructosuria, caused by an autosomal recessive lack of the enzyme fructokinase. This results in spilling abnormal amounts of fructose into the urine. This type of fructosuria is not dangerous and causes no difficulties unless it is misdiagnosed as diabetes mellitus. No treatment is required for this entity.

Some other disorders of carbohydrate metabolism result from derangements in either the synthesis or degradation of glycogen and its subsequent utilization. In most of these illnesses the liver is the principal organ involved, though in some cases the heart can be affected as well, by becoming infiltrated by deposits of glycogen.

Von Gierke and Pompe diseases are two diseases of glycogenosis. Each is characterized by the absence of a specific enzyme in the glycogen metabolism cycle. The most frequent type is von Gierke, which is caused by an absence of the enzyme glucose-6-phosphatase; diagnosis can be accomplished by demonstrated absence of this specific enzyme. Treatment is directed toward preventing hypoglycemia with dietary programs.

Disorders of Lipid Metabolism

The most frequent types of abnormality in lipid metabolism are the hypolipoproteinemias where the major plasma lipids, particularly cholesterol and the triglycerides, are found in excessive quantities. These disorders are frequently genetic, being inherited in either a recessive or dominant fashion. Though they do cause severe disease in adults and can result in early atherosclerosis and coronary heart disease, they do not cause many difficulties in children. Because these are not germane to our discussion of developmental disabilities, they will not be discussed in this book. Information concerning these diseases is readily available from the American Heart Association.

Another group of lipidoses, though rare, can cause serious and severe damage to children by causing an accumulation of abnormal lipids (fats) in the cells and organs of the body.

Gaucher disease   Principal among these diseases is Gaucher disease where there is an accumulation of abnormal glucocerebrosides (complex molecules of sugars and fats) in the reticuloendothelial cells of the body. This usually is manifested clinically by an enlarged liver and spleen accompanied by changes in the pigmentation of the skin. This condition may appear in childhood with an onset in infancy or may occur later in adult life. When occurring in infants, the onset is usually more acute with signs of involvement of the brain. Death in infants usually occurs within a year though those who survive to adolescence may live for many years.

No specific treatment is known, though in cases where there is severe enlargement, splenectomy may be advised.

Niemann-Pick disease is similar in many forms to Gaucher except that it is an accumulation of a different fat, sphingomyelin, in the reticuloendothelial cells. This disease appears most often in Jewish families; treatment is supportive as there is no specific therapy.

Tay-Sachs disease (amaurotic familial idiocy) and related disorders This is a group of disorders which shows an increase in the lipid content of certain tissues particularly the nerve cells in the brain. A number of these disorders have been described to date, and all of them involve abnormalities of specific enzymes necessary in the lipid metabolism of the brain cells.

The three disorders most frequently known and discussed are Tay-Sachs (the early infantile form), Bielschowsky-Jansky disease (the early juvenile form), and Spielmeyer-Vogt disease (the late juvenile form).

Tay-Sachs is the most commonly encountered of these lipid diseases, occurring principally among people of Jewish descent, particularly the Ashkenazic Jewish population coming from eastern Europe. Approximately 10% of the cases of Tay-Sachs may occur in non-Jewish populations. This is a recessive genetic disease, and though quite rare nationally, it does have a significant occurrence rate in this population of Jewish people.

Tay-Sachs usually begins to cause symptoms in children at approximately six months of age. There is a rapid and progressive degeneration of the central nervous system accompanied by severe and profound mental and motor retardation with death usually occurring at two and a half to four years of age. The first symptoms occurring are usually irritability, some vomiting, and a noticeable failure to thrive. Vision becomes noticeably worse, and a small cherry red spot can usually be seen in the macula on the retina of the eye. There is a failure to grow with an ultimate development of severe respiratory problems. There appears to be a deterioration or change in the nerve cells of the brain because of the accumulation of abnormal lipids.

There is no known effective treatment at this time.

Bielschowsky-Jansky disease usually does not manifest itself until three to four years of age. Degeneration is essentially the same as in Tay-Sachs, except that it proceeds at a slower rate.

Spielmeyer-Vogt disease manifests itself usually between the ages of six and eight and continues for ten to twelve years. Symptoms again are those of wasting. The average age at death is 18 years of age. Spielmeyer-Vogt disease is found to occur more frequently in people of northern European stock; the gene responsible for this disease is not the same as that producing Tay-Sachs disease.

Metachromatic leukodystrophy is a progressive central nervous system disease caused by a deficiency of the enzyme cerebroside sulfatase. The lack of this enzyme permits abnormal fats to accumulate in the white matter of the central nervous system, in the peripheral nerves, kidney, spleen, and other visceral organs. It is characterized by progressive paralysis, brain deterioration, and frank dementia on occasions. Onset of the disease is usually at about age two to three and it is fatal by age 11 to 12.

Krabbe disease   This autosomal recessive disease results from a deficiency of another enzyme necessary for metabolism of brain lipids. It is a fatal infantile disorder characterized by progressive retardation, paralysis, blindness, deafness, and palsies. The diagnosis of this disorder may be made prenatally from amniotic fluid. (See final section of Chapter 8.)

MISCELLANEOUS DISEASES

Wilson Disease, Hepatolenticular Degeneration

This is an autosomal recessive disease characterized by degeneration of the brain stem and a breakdown of liver structure. This disorder results from an abnormality in the metabolism of copper, resulting in an accumulation of excessive amounts of copper, particularly in the liver and brain. Its occurrence rate is about one in 4 million live births, so it is extremely rare.

After years of laying down excessive amounts of copper, particularly in the brain, the disease manifests itself with tremors, difficulty in swallowing, and frequently with emotional and mental abnormalities. Dementia or psychotic behavior can occur, resulting in the misdiagnosis of psychotic disease. Treatment can be accomplished if the disease is found early, by reducing copper intake in the diet and by the use of medications which increase the excretion of copper in the urine.

Marfan Syndrome

This is a skeletal and connective tissue disease, resulting in an individual who is tall and thin, with an exceptionally long torso. The face is usually elongated and thin, and the arms are long with very long spidery fingers. It is not infrequent to see a displaced lens in the eyes of these individuals. This condition is inherited as an autosomal dominant trait occurring in about three in 200,000 births in the general population. Mental retardation occurs only rarely with this syndrome. Though there is no treatment indicated except for symptomatic treatment of the eye disorders, these individuals need to be watched carefully for dilatation of the aorta, the large blood vessel coming from the heart, as it frequently dilates and can rupture.

Osteogenesis Imperfecta

This is an inherited disease estimated to occur in between one per 20,000 to one per 60,000 live births. There are two basic forms, the congenital form which occurs and is present at birth, and the tardive type, which is more common and usually much milder, appearing at about the time of puberty.

This disease is inherited as an autosomal dominant trait in the tardive form; the congenital form is probably inherited as a recessive trait. The major difficulties in these children are abnormally formed skeletal structures which sustain numerous fractures, many times with poor healing; mental retardation does not usually accompany this disease.

Until recently, no effective treatment had been known. The recent use of fluorides is under investigation. The fractures are treated in the usual manner with reduction and splinting.

Hurler Syndrome

This syndrome is a group of diseases involving abnormal metabolism of the mucopolysaccharides (gelatinous complex sugar compounds). These are divided into Type I, Hurler; Type II, Hunter; Type III, Sanfilippo; Type IV, Morquio; Type V, Sheie; and Type VI, Maroteaux-Lamy. Though each of these types involves a different enzyme abnormality, they are all caused by abnormal recessive genes that prevent the formation of specific enzymes necessary in the metabolism of the mucopolysaccharides. Almost all tissues and most cells in the body are affected in these diseases. Normal tissue and cell structures are invaded and distorted by the abnormal cells, which appear to contain accumulations of mucopolysaccharides. In all these different types, there are frequent eye disorders with clouding of the cornea, and the children are usually small-statured, if not actually dwarfed.

Hurler syndrome, Type I, is a rare connective tissue disease characterized by severe mental retardation, seizures, blindness, hepatosplenomegaly (enlargement of the liver and spleen), and deformities of the skull and facial bones. It is sometimes called gargoylism because of the abnormally shaped heads and faces.

The Type II variant, Hunter disease, is less severe than Hurler, and while the major clinical manifestations are similar, mental deterioration progresses at a slower rate and the extent of corneal clouding is usually less severe. In Hunter disease, the genetic carrier is located on the X chromosome, so that it is a sex-linked, or X-linked, trait with rare female involvement. The female carrier is unaffected.

There is no specific treatment for either Hurler or Hunter diseases at the present time except for symptomatic treatment of the eye symptoms and seizure difficulties as they occur. Recent trials with cortisone drugs result in some biochemical changes but do not appear to result in any long-term improvement in the disease.

Hydrocephalus

Hydrocephalus is an abnormal accumulation of cerebrospinal fluid within the ventricles (small chambers) of the brain. The cerebrospinal fluid is the fluid formed within the brain which fills the small chambers and bathes the entire brain and spinal cord.

The cerebrospinal fluid is formed by a network of blood vessels called the choroid plexus. There is a delicate balance between the production of fluid by this plexus and its rate of absorption in other areas of the brain. Hydrocephalus occurs when there is an excessive amount of fluid, either due to an overproduction or an underabsorption of fluid, or to obstruction of the normal flow. This rapid accumulation distends and dilates the ventricles, causing pressure on the cerebral cortex and other parts of the brain. If it is not relieved, it will cause damage to the cells in the brain. An obstruction can occur in many locations of the ventricular system, and the extent of the hydrocephalus and its location will depend on where the obstruction occurs.

The communicating, or infantile, type of hydrocephalus is usually due to a faulty absorption of the cerebrospinal fluid and not due to obstruction in the ventricles.

An infant developing hydrocephalus after birth shows a tense, bulging fontanel, or "soft spot." Because of the increased pressure, the child is usually irritable and frightened. Vomiting is an early symptom. A rapidly enlarging head, by measurement, is usually indicative of hydrocephalus.

Treatment is principally surgical, with the insertion of a plastic tube into the ventricle of the brain which then shunts the cerebrospinal fluid through a valve into the abdomen where it is absorbed. Treatment of this type of disease, if diagnosed early, has been excellent, and children will usually progress with a minimal amount of brain damage.

Neural Tube Defects

The nervous system develops very early in the embryo's life (within the first few weeks). First it is like an almost flat plate, but it will round up and fuse. This fusion begins almost in the middle and extends both toward tail and toward the head of the embryo. If there is a failure in the normal embryologic growth, there can be a lack of fusion on one end or the other with resultant physical abnormalities in the child.

Spina bifida is caused by a failure of the vertebral arches to unite in the midline. It usually occurs just above the buttocks. The extent of the spina bifida can be minimal with nothing more than a simple dimple, and perhaps, a bony defect being noted on x-ray. There may be no physical difficulties and the child, for all intents and purposes, grows and develops normally. Larger defects can cause a protrusion of the linings, or meninges, of the spinal cord, causing a meningocele. Still more serious defects may take the form of a protrusion, or herniation, of the spinal cord into the spina bifida; this is called a meningomyelocele.

Children with a meningomyelocele can have severe difficulties, as it can damage or totally disrupt the nervous system control to the lower legs, buttocks, and genitalia. Paralysis may be partial or complete, and there may be partial or complete absence of sphincter control of the bladder and bowels.

Treatment will depend upon the extent of the damage; in some cases some surgical treatment might be indicated.

Encephalocele is a defect at the other end of the cord occurring in the region of the head. These defects are present at birth. They are usually in the midline on the lower back of the head, or the occiput. Attempts in treating these are difficult, and the ultimate outlook is usually poor.

Hydrocephalus is frequently associated with neural tube defects and must be evaluated in each child.

The most serious of the neural tube defects is a total anencephaly where there is a failure of the brain to form. Here, lower centers of the brain only might develop, with no development of the cerebral cortex. These children usually do not live more than a few hours or days.

Neural tube defects are polygenic genetic diseases with a risk of recurrence of 5% to 7% in future children.

Parents having one child with a neural tube defect should seek genetic counseling in regard to future pregnancies and the possibility of diagnosing any subsequent children prenatally.

Laurence-Moon-Biedl Syndrome

This syndrome is a recessive hereditary disorder characterized by five main symptoms: 1) polydactylism (extra fingers and toes on an extremity), 2) obesity, 3) hypogonadism (poorly developed genitals), 4) retinitis pigmentosa, and 5) usually moderate to severe mental retardation.

Retinitis pigmentosa, which may occur in other diseases, is a degenerative inflammatory condition involving excessive pigmentation in the retina of the eye. It appears usually between six and fourteen years of age and shows increasing pigment with resultant loss in night vision at first. As the condition progresses, visual fields become narrowed, and these people can develop tunnel vision or total blindness in certain cases.

The obesity is one of the most marked, obvious symptoms. It is felt that this is due to a basic defect in the brain permitting the development of severe hunger; appetites may be enormous.

There is no specific treatment for the syndrome as a whole. The extra fingers and toes and the webbing between the fingers and toes can be corrected surgically, and the obesity can be controlled by careful dieting programs. Investigations using surgical procedures as treatment are currently underway; no data are available as yet.

Cornelia de Lange Syndrome

This is a syndrome consisting of severe mental retardation coupled with specific multiple anomalies of the face and the extremities. Various estimates of the incidence of this disorder place it between one per 10,000 and one per 100,000 births with the probable figure being about one in 60,000 to 75,000. The etiology is unknown, though there is some suggestive evidence that this is a recessive autosomal genetic trait.

Infants born with the Cornelia de Lange syndrome usually are small-for-date infants weighing less than five and a half pounds at birth, and they show continued mental and motor retardation throughout life. They frequently have extensive hirsutism, particularly with hairiness of the eyebrows and eyelashes. The head is usually small and disproportionately short, the nasal bridge is depressed, and the nostrils turned forward. The lips are usually thin and turned down at the corners giving them a "carplike" appearance.

Deformities of the extremities can be extreme. Limited movement in the elbows occurs, and an abnormal location of the thumb is common, being located higher on the wrists than normal. Webbing between the fingers and toes is frequent.

These children may also show congenital hip dislocations, delayed bone maturation, and delayed maturity of secondary sexual characteristics. These children can be extremely restless, destructive, and self-mutilating. Epilepsy is a frequent complicating problem. There is no specific treatment for this condition, but specific therapy for the orthopedic deformities may be undertaken.

Lesch-Nyhan Syndrome

This syndrome is an inborn error involving an abnormality of uric acid metabolism. These children have severe global retardation in both motor and intellectual spheres. They present with findings resembling spastic cerebral palsy, and develop severe self-mutilating behavior—biting their fingers, toes, and lips.

134

This disease is transmitted as an X-linked recessive where the defective gene is on the X female chromosome. The carrier mother will show no signs of the disease, but 50% of her male offspring will have this disease.

The diagnosis can be conclusively established by metabolic chemical determinations of the child's blood. Height and weight are usually far below normal. The self-mutilating behavior can be severe and, though the children feel pain, they will mutilate themselves in spite of it. They will frequently request that an observer prevent them from mutilating themselves, because of the pain involved.

Treatment has not evolved at this time, though experimental work is currently underway in evaluating the use of some of the medications that interfere with or enhance the uric acid metabolism.

Tuberous Sclerosis

Tuberous sclerosis is a disorder in which tumorlike masses are found in many different organs in the body. They cause mental retardation principally by involving areas in the brain, destroying functioning brain tissue. These tumorlike masses (tubers) in the brain tend to enlarge, produce epileptic seizures, and impair brain function in the process of their growth. Similar lesions can occur in the sweat glands and present the most obvious signs consisting of small growths on the nose, cheek, and lip areas. Epilepsy, mental retardation, and sebaceous adenoma (the small tumors on the nose) are highly suggestive of tuberous sclerosis.

Tuberous sclerosis occurs equally in males and females, in about one in 150,000 births. There is a marked variation in the "expression" of the disease, and many members of the family will be affected differently—one child severely retarded, another child or parent with nothing more than small adenomas on their nose.

Diagnosis is usually made by finding the classic triad of symptoms, epilepsy, sebaceous adenoma, and mental retardation, and frequently by finding deposits of calcium in the areas of the brain tumors. This triad of symptoms is usually not present at birth, and each of the three symptoms may evolve at different developmental ages. Epilepsy frequently makes its appearance at approximately two years of age. The sebaceous adenomas commonly appear between ages two and six, and mental retardation is the last to be definitely diagnosed. Persons with tuberous sclerosis not having any brain lesions may have normal intellectual abilities. Treatment consists of controlling the symptomatology and the epilepsy if it occurs. Little can be done to treat the skin lesions or the lesions in the brain.

Neurofibromatosis or von Recklinghausen Disease

This disease presents in many respects like tuberous sclerosis. Multiple benign tumors occur in the brain, spinal canal, and skin. The frequency of epilepsy is much less than in tuberous sclerosis.

The incidence of neurofibromatosis is about one in 2000 and is usually transmitted in a dominant inherited fashion. Here again, there is a marked variation in the severity. One family member may have thousands of neurofibromas involving his skin, another member may show nothing more than a café au lait (brown) spot on the skin.

Damage is caused by the growth of the tumors where they exert pressure on the nervous system, either in the brain or along the spinal cord. No specific treatment is available for the basic disease process.

Sturge-Weber Syndrome

This disease is a dominant genetic disorder characterized by a "port wine stain" (venous angioma) in the membrane surrounding the brain on one side. There is usually a port wine stain on the same side of the face and neck as the angioma occurring in the brain. Calcium deposits may occur on this same side of the brain leading to mental retardation and paralysis of the opposite side of the body. Findings of this syndrome are extremely variable because of the extent of the involvement of the brain. Epilepsy, if it occurs, usually occurs early during the first year of life in the form of a unilateral seizure occurring on the side opposite the angioma. The patient may have a relatively normal mental development during the first few months of life and may or may not become progressively retarded. There is usually no relationship between the severity of the lesion on the face and the severity of the intercranial lesion or resultant retardation. Occasionally, abnormalities of the eyes are noted.

The only form of treatment is surgical removal of the affected area of the brain if this can be accomplished. Surgical treatment is rather new and is presently being evaluated as to its long-term effectiveness. Treatment, otherwise, is purely symptomatic in treating the seizure disorder and cosmetic care of the port wine angioma.

Achondroplasia

This is the most common of the chondrodystrophies, a group of diseases which result in deformities of the development of the skeletal system. It is in this general group of diseases that most dwarfs occur.

Achondroplasia is a dominant genetic disease, though most cases present as new mutations. Paternal age appears to play a causative role, as there is an increased incidence of achondroplasia occurring with older fathers. These children are usually diagnosable at birth. They have an enlarged, prominent forehead, stubby arms and legs, and frequently hydrocephalus.

The extremities are short, but the trunk may be normal in size with the proximal (closer to the body) bones being more involved than the bones on the ends of the extremities.

Mental retardation usually is not present but may appear secondary to the hydrocephalus, the increased cranial pressure causing damage to the brain, if not treated and relieved. Motor development is usually delayed until approximately two years of age.

Apert Syndrome (Acrocephalosyndactyly)

Children with this syndrome have an early fusion (craniostenosis) of the coronal sutures of the head resulting in a lengthening of the head vertically. They have a characteristic facial appearance, a small maxilla and prominent eyes, widely spaced. Frequently they have fusion of the hands with involvement of the thumbs and toes.

Mental retardation occurs with varying degrees of severity which may vary from minor to profound.

Ataxia Telangiectasia (Louis-Bar Syndrome)

These children have frequent telangiectasia, or blood vessel tumors, which affect mainly the face, ears, neck, hands, wrists, and knees. They frequently have telangiectasia (blood-vessel tumors) of the conjunctiva of the eye, usually appearing by age three to four. These telangiectasias can also occur in the brain and, if present, cause brain damage usually to the cerebrum. This damage causes difficulty in balance and walking.

Frequently the immune system is absent or abnormal; infections are frequent. Mental retardation occurs in approximately one-third of the patients, usually late in the disease as a result of the neurologic involvement.

Congenital Hypothyroidism (Cretinism)

Cretinism occurs in approximately one in 5000 births in the United States and it is only recently that general screening is being done in most states for this disease. If untreated, the child can show severe retardation, which will vary with the degree of the disease and also the age at diagnosis. Children not diagnosed until a late age are almost uniformly severely retarded.

These children have delayed skeletal maturation; dry, cold extremities; puffiness about their eyes; and a characteristic facial appearance of a large tongue protruding from the open mouth. They have frequent respiratory difficulties with marked difficulty in breathing, secondary to the large tongue. They usually have a prominent abdomen; umbilical hernias are frequent. Their hair is coarse and brittle. The children are usually quite hypotonic with marked delay in motor development.

Diagnosis is accomplished by standard thyroid function tests which can be done during the newborn period. Treatment using thyroid hormone, if instituted early, is usually very effective.

MATERNAL INFECTIONS

Maternal infections play an important role in the causation of mental retardation, as many infections can be transmitted from the mother to the fetus through the placenta or to the fetus during its passage through the birth canal during labor. These infections can cause severe to extensive damage depending upon the time of gestation that the infection occurs and the organ systems involved by the infective agent.

Congenital Rubella

Rubella, or German measles, is an acute contagious disease most often seen in children, and is caused by a virus. Rubella in most children, though it may cause acute febrile symptoms, is usually relatively benign, except in the rare case of a complicating infection or a complicating encephalomyelitis. Rubella occurring in the mother, however, can have severe consequences if it occurs during the early embryologic development stage of the embryo (during the first trimester of pregnancy). Research has indicated that if acute infection occurs during this time, malformations will occur in from 20% to 80% of the infants.

Early reports indicated that if rubella occurred after the fourth month of pregnancy there were no difficulties. Recently the possibility has been raised that this late infection might be a cause of mental retardation without other physical defects. This is being researched.

Infections occurring in the pregnancy can cause damage severe enough to result in stillbirth or spontaneous abortion. Nonfatal infection with a rubella virus is known to cause cataracts, heart defects, deafness, glaucoma, and certain defects of the teeth. The virus is known to be harbored in the child and can be cultured from the child for several weeks to months after delivery. Whether this results in any long-term, slowly progressive central nervous system damage is not clearly understood at this time. The virus causes its damage by actually invading the different body cells. The cells most typically invaded are those of the brain, heart, eyes, and ears.

Diagnosis is determined by either isolating the virus from an affected child or in finding high rubella titers in a fetus whose mother has had a proven case of rubella during her pregnancy. Antibody titers can be determined in the mother, and any mother suspected of having acute rubella infections should be tested to see if her antibody titer increases between the beginning and the end of this acute infection.

There is no specific treatment for this disease except for supportive treatment where indicated. Congenital heart disease can be repaired in most cases surgically, and cataracts can frequently be helped with surgical intervention. In some situations where the mother is in her first trimester, a therapeutic abortion might be considered.

Congenital Syphilis

Congenital syphilis has become a relatively rare disease in the United States in recent years. With the recent upsurge in reported cases of syphilis, however, it is anticipated that this disease could once again increase in frequency. These children present with abnormalities at birth with frequent rhinitis, or sniffles, and nasal obstruction. The liver and spleen are frequently enlarged, the children are anemic, and jaundice is an early manifestation. They can have an inflammation of the retina and iris of the eyes, and the skin will frequently show rashes with predilection for occurrence on the buttocks and posterior thighs. Inflammations involving the skeletal structure with an osteochondritis (an inflammation) involving the wrists, ankles, and knees are quite common. Untreated cases can develop meningitis, muscle-wasting disease, and hydrocephaly. Late manifestations can include severe brain damage with paralysis and seizures. Diagnosis is accomplished by finding positive serology for syphilis. Treatment is accomplished with penicillin or other antibiotics.

Toxoplasmosis

Toxoplasmosis is an infection caused by the protozoa *Toxoplasma gondii.* This infection in the infant is usually acquired by travel of the protozoa across the placenta to infect the embryo, the mother presumably having acquired an infection shortly before or during pregnancy. If infection occurs early in pregnancy, a spontaneous abortion can occur. Severe infection later in the pregnancy can result in miscarriage or stillbirth.

The disease may present in the infant in many forms. It may be severe, fulminating, and rapidly fatal, or it may show no symptoms at all. The most frequent symptoms are severe jaundice with enlargement of the liver and spleen, a skin rash, and chorioretinitis, an infection of the eye. Convulsions are frequent with this disease when there is central nervous system involvement; small areas of infection can ultimately lead to calcification which can be found on x-rays in older children. Severe involvement of the eye can lead to blindness, and extensive involvement of the brain can lead to mild to severe mental retardation.

The diagnosis can be made by antibody tests of the mother's and the baby's bloods. The prognosis is generally poor for the acute neonatal form of congenital toxoplasmosis, because of the severe destructive brain lesions. There is a form of postnatal acquired infection which apparently runs a rather mild course. This disease is rarely fatal.

There is no known treatment for the chronic congenital lesions, but treatment of the acute form in adults can be accomplished with medications.

Cytomegalic Inclusion Disease

This is an infection that can occur congenitally, postnatally, or at any time later in life. It ranges in severity from a silent infection without consequences through a severe infection causing extensive brain damage, resulting in stillbirth or perinatal death in the fetus.

The cytomegaloviruses are known as the salivary gland viruses and are quite similar to the herpes group of viruses. Following an infection, individuals may excrete this virus in the urine or saliva for many months, and it can be found in the urine of infected infants. It is a frequent infection, and 60% to 90% of adults have experienced an infection with this type of virus at some time during their lives.

In congenital infections the extent of the disease is highly variable. It might be found only by demonstrating the virus in the urine of an otherwise apparently normal infant, or it may go to the other extreme, showing severe central nervous system infection with resultant abortion or stillbirth. Children born with the severe form of the disease usually have a low birthweight, frequently develop a fever after being born, and show evidence of liver infection. There can be involvement of the eye, and damage to the central nervous system can result in microcephaly with severe retardation, blindness, deafness, or seizures. Hearing defects may be manifest in children with severe disease. There is no specific therapy for this disease, and the results of recent trials with some of the newer antiviral drugs have not been conclusive as to their efficacy.

Herpes

There are at least two strains of known herpes viruses. Type I causes the herpes simplex seen about the lips and is commonly called cold sores or fever blisters. Type II is usually genital and may be transmitted venereally.

Herpes simplex, Type I, usually does not cause any infections that create problems in young infants and children except for the casual cold sore or fever blister occurring in almost all people.

Type II, however, is increasing in frequency and is becoming a frequent cause of severe fulminating infection in the newborn. The Type II virus is moderately contagious and is usually spread in adults by sexual intercourse. Lesions usually develop in women on the labia, clitoris, perineum, vagina, and may be present on the cervix. They tend to heal spontaneously only to recur without a specific instigating cause.

In the newborn, herpes can cause severe disease if there is an acute infection occurring at or near the time of delivery, as the virus appears to invade the infant as the baby passes through an infected birth canal. For this reason, caesarean section at term, before the membranes have ruptured, is the delivery method of choice to prevent exposure of the infant to this virus.

Infants infected with this virus usually develop a severe central nervous system encephalitis which, until recently, has been almost uniformly fatal. New antiviral medications have been used in the past few years with some success in preventing mortality. But the children so treated are not yet old enough to determine the extent of central nervous system damage which might have occurred.

12 Down Syndrome

In 1866, John Langdon Down, a physician in England, published the first comprehensive description of what we know as Down syndrome. His clinical description at that time is still quite accurate today. Because of a fairly typical appearance of the faces of these children, he called them "Mongols." Unfortunately, the term mongolism became quite widely used, being used by Down himself. It was Down's opinion that these children resembled the Mongolian race. This, of course, is an unfortunate and inappropriate choice because there is a suggestion of racial origin, which is totally incorrect.

Many people feel that the term "Down syndrome" is an unscientific name for the age-old problem of mongolism. At the time Down described this syndrome, he perceived correctly that an unusual biologic phenomenon was occurring in these children. His scheme for an ethnic classification of retarded children, or idiots as they were called in those days, was in harmony with the contemporary scientific thought that had been influenced by Darwin's theories of evolution. The ethnic theory never became very popular, but the term Mongol came into general use and has continued up until recent time. Down's concept of a reversion to early phylogenic type was supported as late as 1924 by Cruickshank, who felt that this was regression to a more primitive Oriental human type. These concepts, of course, were unfounded and are no longer referred to in any literature.

Today we know that this condition results from a chromosome abnormality, there being an extra No. 21 chromosome. For this reason, Down syndrome is frequently called trisomy-21. Down syndrome occurs in all races, in all walks of life, in all areas of social environment. It has even been reported in some of the great apes, particularly the orangutans. Even though the chromosomal abnormalities associated with Down syndrome are well described, the actual cause of the disease is unknown. The

142

underlying cause appears to be a nondisjunction, or a failure of the chromosomes to separate during the formation of the sex cells (the sperm and/or the egg). In approximately 92% of cases, the cause appears to be a straight nondisjunction with a resultant extra No. 21 chromosome giving a chromosome count of 47 instead of the usual number of 46. (See Figure 12-1.)

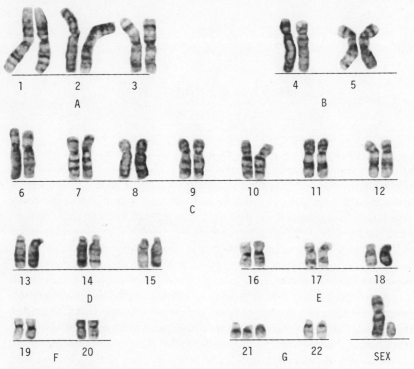

Figure 12-1 Karyotype of a Down syndrome child, 47 XY + 21.

Approximately 5% of Down syndrome patients show the normal number, 46; however, the morphology may be altered due to a translocation. In a translocation, an extra No. 21 chormosome may be attached to either one of the coexisting No. 21 chromosomes or to a chromosome from another group, usually the No. 14 or 15. These aberrations may be due to spontaneous or inherited translocations. Figure 12-2 shows a translocation in a Down syndrome patient.

Because of a possibility of translocation, all children suspected of having Down syndrome should have a karyotype to be sure that they are not carrying a translocated 21 chormosome. If these children do have a translocation, both their parents should also have a karyotype to find out whether they are carriers. Balanced carriers have the right complement of chromosomes and therefore the correct amount of DNA in their cells.

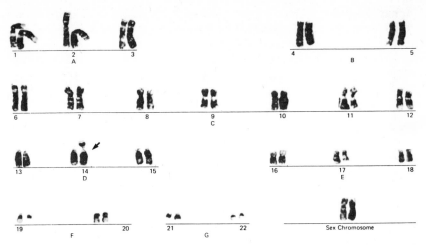

Figure 12-2   Translocation in a Down syndrome patient.

However, they have a 50% chance of transmitting the translocated abnormal chromosome to any sex cells they might produce and a 30% chance of another Down infant. The other 20% of Down fetuses are probably aborted spontaneously.

The third type of Down syndrome seen in 2% to 5% of cases is called mosaicism. Mosaicism occurs when two cell populations coexist in the same individual. In these cases, some of the cells of the individual will have the normal complement of 46 chromosomes and some of the cells will have a complement of 47 chromosomes. People having mosaic Down syndrome show all the phenotypic (physical) stigmata of the disease, though perhaps to a lesser extent than those children with straight trisomy-21 or a translocation Down syndrome.

To date, the reason for the failure of separation of the chromosomes in the gametes (the egg or sperm) is unknown. One well-established fact is that older maternal age is associated with increased risk of having a baby with Down syndrome. At the present time, increased paternal age has not been shown to be a causative factor.

The occurrence rate of Down syndrome is approximately one in every 700 to 750 live births. In women age 21 to 27, the risk is approximately one in 1500 and remains quite low until age 35. At this time the risk increases rapidly, reaching a risk of 2% at age 40. (See Figure 12-3.)

It is important that a mother having a Down child be assured that there is nothing that "went wrong" during her pregnancy. Nothing she ate or did, no medication taken, or any other activity could have caused this defect. The event that produced Down syndrome occurred either at or before the time of conception.

The Down syndrome child can frequently be diagnosed clinically at birth. There are instances, however, where we have seen Down children

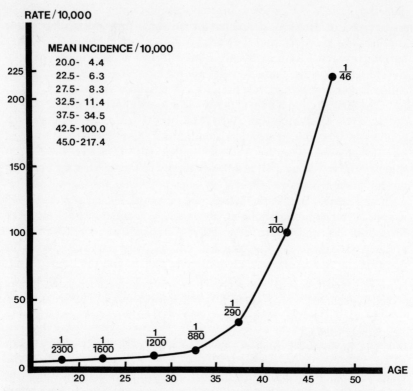

RATE/10,000

MEAN INCIDENCE / 10,000

20.0-	4.4
22.5-	6.3
27.5-	8.3
32.5-	11.4
37.5-	34.5
42.5-	100.0
45.0-	217.4

Figure 12-3 Incidence of Down syndrome as related to maternal age. Adapted from: Coleman, R.D., and Stoller, A. Notes on the epidemiology of monogolism in Victoria, Australia from 1942 to 1957. Proc. Lond. Conf. Study Mental Def. 2, 517; and Mikkelsen, M., and Stene, J. Genetic Counseling in Down's syndrome. *Human Heredity* 20:457–464, 1970.

who appear quite normal in the nursery, and there are instances when children have the appearance of Down syndrome but have a normal karyotype and turn out to be normal children.

We recently saw a 34-year-old woman who was diagnosed as being a "Mongol" when she was born. At that time, there were no karyotyping studies able to make a definitive diagnosis. It was not until just recently, when she came to us for evaluation and premarital consultation, that a karyotype was done, and she was found to be perfectly normal. This woman had lived under the stigma of being labeled a mongoloid for 34 years and had foregone marriage and any consideration of a family until this late stage of her life.

The definitive diagnosis must be made by performing a chromosomal karyotype which involves looking at the chromosomes microscopically, determining the exact number of chromosomes and their morphology. This was described in Chapter 9.

Perhaps one of the more interesting things about Down syndrome, is that the extra No. 21 chromosome confers upon these children a phenotypic, or physical, characteristic in which they are similar to one another—far more so than they are similar to their parents. True, they have their parents' skin, hair, eye color, but their general facial features, stature, and physical characteristics are far more characteristic of Down children as a group than they are of their individual parents.

The features that make up the syndrome are apparently conferred by the extra No. 21 chromosome. Why this little extra piece of DNA material confers this phenotypic response is unknown. These children have typical physical characteristics, yet they are individuals. Typically, the child is short-statured, has a small head, is mentally retarded. He may have abnormal facial features, a guttural cry when born, and poor startle reflexes normally present in infants. Muscle tone is poor. The head is small and rounded with some flattening at the back, the tongue is rather large for the mouth and tends to protrude. There is frequently an excessive fat pad at the nape of the neck and frequently a single transverse crease across the palm of the hand—the so-called "simian" line. The joints are hypermobile. There are frequent findings of other congenital defects, particularly heart disease, cleft lip and palate, and bowel abnormalities. In infancy there is a high incidence of acute leukemia.

The ultimate intellectual capacity of the child is impossible to ascertain early in life. Down children can be extremely retarded with IQs as low as 20, but some have been reported to have IQs as high as 90 or 92. Current early intervention programs used in recent years appear to elevate the ultimate intellectual capacity of these children. These intervention programs are designed to stimulate children and help them obtain their full potential for social, emotional, physical, and cognitive growth. These programs follow specific patterns of development and are designed to stimulate motor activities, language activities, social and emotional behavior.

Down children usually make slow, steady progress as normal children do. If developmental curves are followed, they are found to progress fairly normally during the first three to four months, and then to fall behind other children. They have some delay in sitting, standing, walking, and speech is almost always delayed. Progress cannot be forecast in any one given child, and the ultimate development depends upon inherited variables and the input of well-developed and founded intervention and educational programs. Approximately 2% to 4% of these children will have IQs that reach into the low normal range.

ASSOCIATED CONGENITAL DEFECTS

Children with Down syndrome have frequent congenital defects. Congenital heart disease is common, and incidence figures have been

146

reported to vary from 7.1% to 64.2 % with an average of 19%. The defects are varied. Some are severe being incompatible with life; others require nothing more than careful watching. The majority of congenital heart defects are amenable to surgery, and the child should be referred early to a cardiologist for evaluation, diagnosis, and possible surgery.

Cleft palate and harelip occur in about 0.5% of children with Down syndrome, considerably higher than in the general population.

The tongue, though normal at birth, usually later develops some hypertrophy or enlargement of some of the papillae. As the child becomes older, it is common to see some fissuring in the tongue.

Teething is frequently delayed; the teeth are frequently abnormally shaped, and some of the deciduous, or baby teeth, may be absent. The permanent teeth may also be delayed, though they tend to appear more regularly. The teeth appear to be small and show abnormalities in shape, such as being peg-shaped or having some malformations on the crown; malocclusion is frequently reported. The dental problems are amenable to treatment in most cases; the child usually has minimal caries for his age group if proper dental hygiene is maintained.

The eyes show an oblique and narrow palpebral fissure, or opening, particularly in a young child. There is a tendency for them to slant upward in infancy and youth, though adults' eyes tend to be more horizontal. An epicanthic fold, or flap, on the inside of the eye is very common, being reported in as high as 80% of cases. Visual difficulties are frequent, either due to difficulty with eye muscle movement or, in some cases, to opacities within the lens. Strabismus, myopia, hyperopia, nystagmus, and cataracts are frequently seen. Most of these conditions are treatable, and the child should be examined by a competent ophthalmologist early in life if there appears to be any difficulty.

The child with Down syndrome tends to have a distended, prominent abdomen. This is probably related to the general hypotonia. Umbilical hernias are frequent, reported in 12% to 15% of the children.

There are frequent abnormalities in the intestinal tract, and there is an association of Hirschsprung disease, or megacolon, on occasion. Constipation in Down children is a frequent complaint of parents and can usually be treated with routine measures.

Upon reaching adulthood, Down syndrome people are usually short in stature. Their hands are chunky, but they have no motor defects and, except for coordination problems, are capable of almost any type of normal body movement.

Sexual development might be late in onset or incomplete or both. Males tend to produce less testosterone and may have relatively small penis and less facial hair than usual. Females have mild to moderate breast development, and menstruation is usually delayed two to three years. Sexual drives are usually diminished, though a few women with Down syndrome have reproduced; approximately 50% of their offspring have had Down syndrome. No man with Down syndrome has ever been recorded as having fathered a child. It is presumed that they are infertile.

As children, Down syndrome patients have frequent and chronic infections, particularly of the respiratory tract. They have recurrent tonsilitis, ear infections, bronchitis, and pneumonias. During the first five years of the children's lives, most mothers become totally frustrated with the frequent infections. It seems that they are always going to the doctor because their youngsters are sick. Hope does spring on the the horizon for these parents, as the majority of the children appear to develop better immunity and their frequency of illness decreases quite markedly after they reach age five. In years past, prior to the advent of antibiotics, the vast majority of these children died during infancy from a severe infection, particularly pneumonia. Today, this is no longer critical if they are treated adequately and frequently. The actual defect in the immune system has not been described, but there appears to be difficulty in either developing or utilizing the antibodies normally produced by the body in response to infection.

The majority of Down children are extremely happy, loving children. They are playful and, as a rule, quite easy to manage. It must be remembered that they are subject to the same emotional upsets, and even emotional or psychologic disease occurring in other children. Each one of these problems must be evaluated individually and treated the same as in any other child with a similar emotional disease or complaint.

In years past, the Down child was usually institutionalized, if not immediately after birth, within the first few years. Today, the reverse is true. Institutionalization is rare and only required when home care is not available or in case the child develops severe emotional or psychotic behavior (a rarity). Foster home or family care is usually recommended if it is impossible to maintain the child in the home of his parents. Institutionalization probably potentiates mental retardation rather than helping correct or utilize what intellectual capacities are present. At the age of 18, transition to out-of-home care might include foster or group living homes.

Family Response

It is imperative that parents develop an early positive attitude toward the child. It is important that they exhibit truthfulness, not only to themselves, but to other members of the family. The realization that there is a mentally retarded child in the home can be a very devastating experience. It is, however, important to accept this child as another human being.

After the initial shock, the vast majority of parents of Down children rarely complain of caring for their child in their home; they are happy, loving children, sensitive to a wide range of emotional responses. They will respond to love and attention, and they have capabilities of being taught. The extent of their learning will depend entirely upon the basic intelligence with which they are born.

It is important, however, to stimulate this intelligence to the widest range of its capacity, for if it is not stimulated effectively and early in life, it will become dormant and the child will never reach his ultimate capacity as an adult.

There are three Rs suggested by Dr Richard Koch at the Children's Hospital in Los Angeles for the parent of the retarded child. These are Routine, Relaxation, Repetition.

These children are slower to learn, and it is necessary to establish a specific routine; otherwise they become confused at the variation and variability in activities and stimulations surrounding them.

The parents must be relaxed when they are attempting to train the child and must not be impatient or too expectant. Impatience is not comprehended by these children, and they will progress much more rapidly in an atmosphere of relaxation.

Because the child will respond more slowly, repetition and repetition and repetition are the hallmarks of training and education. If repetition on a specific program is not effective, it is imperative that an alternate plan be attempted to reach this same or, perhaps temporarily, a different goal. We find at many times children do not appear to be ready for certain specific approaches to training, and when they exhibit resistance, a return to a more basic principle or an approach from a different direction is frequently effective in accomplishing the training desired.

Community Facilities

At the present time, there is an enlarging development of multidiscipline team approaches in establishing treatment, training, and intervention programs for the mentally retarded. If these programs are available to parents of handicapped children, they should be utilized in obtaining evaluation and treatment. If such help is not available in the reader's geographic area, there are parent organizations and service agencies available throughout the country. These agencies and organizations can help the parent find diagnostic and intervention programs.

The Exceptional Child Center at Utah State University is part of the nationwide network of University Affiliated Facilities of which there are now over 40 and several satellite programs currently being developed. All these centers are established for the purpose of developing programs of diagnosis, treatment, training, and educational programs for the developmentally disabled child.

Local service agencies and local organizations for the handicapped, are listed in Appendix 2 by general need and by state department or regional clinic concerned. These can be a resource to help parents seek aid.

If all else fails and there is no source of help, any one of the authors will try to secure the help needed for a child. We will be most happy to try to direct people to any of their local resources or to refer them to regional centers.

The multidisciplinary staffs usually include the disciplines of medicine, physical therapy, speech therapy, occupational therapy, psychology, special education, and occasionally dentistry. It is not necessary that all members of this team be working with the child at all times, but when specific problems arise and as the child progresses into new areas of experience, different members of the team might be required to give the parents needed support.

Emotional upsets are not uncommon in parents of retarded children. The situation is stressful, it creates worry; and above all, it creates the question, "Why me?" If the stresses of raising a retarded child become excessive, it is important that the parents seek help and counseling. The situation might be serious enough to require comprehensive counseling by a psychiatrist. If less severe, it might be possible to seek help from a local mental health clinic, local pastor or minister, or from a pediatrician or family physician. It is important not to hesitate to seek help if it becomes necessary—*seek it early.*

The divorce rate in families with a handicapped child is extremely high. Many of these divorces could be prevented if counsel and help were sought early before the conflicts became major. It is imperative that husband and wife develop an open communication between themselves, as a communication deficiency appears to be the most frequent precipitating event causing family disputes.

The problem frequently arises concerning the placement of children with Down syndrome. Most workers in the field today feel that living at home results in the best development for these children. If, for a variety of reasons, this is impossible, the next best solution is to raise the child in a foster home. This home atmosphere, combined with early intervention programs and educational techniques, can result in an intelligence quotient (IQ) 20 to 30 points higher than that found in Down children placed in institutions. With these increasing IQs the children will become better prepared for the life they face in the future.

Today more community facilities are available, as well as improved educational settings designed specifically for the retarded child. These permit him to utilize and develop his intellectual capacities to the fullest. The vast majority of children with Down syndrome can become useful citizens and function quite well at simple, uncomplicated household tasks or within a sheltered workshop program.

Life expectancy in individuals with Down syndrome today approximates 40 or 50 years of age.

Whether Down syndrome adults are increasingly susceptible to certain chronic diseases, tumors, and malignancies is unknown at the present time. Data are being accumulated but are extremely sketchy. It is important during adult life that Down syndrome people have routine physical examinations and evaluations, that their symptoms be carefully evaluated and treated, and that they receive the benefits of good medical care.

At the present time there is no specific treatment for Down syndrome; neither medication nor drugs appear to be effective. Intervention programs and educational programs, both in the home and school, are the major modalities of therapy. Various programs of vitamin therapy and medication therapy have been promulgated in the past, but data to date have not been supportive of any effective results of these programs.

There has been some recent literature on the use of plastic surgery on Down children. At the present time, this is undergoing considerable debate. Certainly, surgical or plastic repair of any obvious defects such as congenital heart defect or cleft lip and palate should be performed. The plastic correction of the flattened nose, the epicanthic fold, the short chin, and other facial characteristics may be indicated in certain specific circumstances. Plastic surgery is expensive, and as cosmetic surgery it is usually not covered by insurance policies. Any corrective surgery must wait until the child is of sufficient size to prevent needless surgical repetition as the child grows older. Decisions concerning plastic surgery must be made on an individual basis and should be made in consultation with a physician.

PREVENTION

Perhaps the biggest inroads possible into the problem of Down syndrome lie with the prevention of the disease. The biggest preventive factor is to encourage women to have their children, if at all possible, before the age of 35.

Women contemplating pregnancy in their late 30s or 40s should realize that there is a risk. To place the risk factors the other way, however, the chances are 95% to 98% that they will not have a baby with Down syndrome. Every woman over age 35, however, should be advised of the availability of amniocentesis with prenatal diagnosis (see Chapter 8). Also, every young woman who has one Down child should be advised concerning the availability of amniocentesis in future pregnancies. Decision to terminate a pregnancy with a Down syndrome is one which the mother and father involved should make, though consultation can be offered by their physician, minister, or genetic counselor.

It is important that parents of children with Down syndrome realize that even though this disease is genetic, the problem is not inherited through the family except, perhaps, in those cases with a translocation chromosome abnormality. There are a few families in which the incidence of Down syndrome seems to be higher than would be anticipated, particularly an increased occurrence in cousins. Why this occurs we do not know at this time. Except in those cases where a translocation is known to exist in the family, chromosome studies need not be done in brothers and sisters of a child with Down syndrome. If there is a translocation in the family, a genetic counselor will need to advise other relatives as to the advisability and necessity of chromosome studies.

In years past, the woman was generally thought to be the cause of the Down child because of the aging of the egg. However, recent techniques have made it possible, in some cases, to determine whether the additional chromosome comes from the father or the mother. Recent studies by R.E. Magenis at the University of Oregon have demonstrated that the mother is not always at fault. He has reported that in approximately 23% of the cases studied, the source of the extra chromosome was the father. It is not always possible to accomplish these special studies, so the test may not always provide an answer. The important point is to know that either the sperm or the egg can be defective in containing an extra chromosome from a nondisjunction.

Pregnant women younger than 35 will frequently ask about prenatal diagnosis for Down syndrome. The relative risks are small, and the costs of amniocentesis average approximately $500 in the United States. Most centers doing these studies would advise that amniocentesis is not indicated in a normal young woman having no history of chromosomal abnormality but would not object to doing it if requested. Most workers in the field agree that the patient should be presented sufficient facts to make an intelligent decision and should choose for themselves instead of leaving this decision to someone else.

13 Cerebral Palsy

Cerebral palsy is a syndrome complex referring to motor disability caused by central nervous system or brain damage. The American Academy of Cerebral Palsy defines the disease as "any abnormal alteration of movement or motor function arising from defect, injury, or disease of the nervous tissues contained in the cranial cavity."

Perhaps a more inclusive definition is that proposed by the United Cerebral Palsy Research and Educational Foundation:

> Cerebral palsy embraces the clinical picture created by injury to the brain in which one of the components is motor disturbance. Thus, cerebral palsy may be described as a group of conditions, usually originating in childhood, characterized by paralysis, weakness, incoordination, or any other aberration of motor function caused by pathology of the motor control center of the brain. In addition to such motor dysfunction, cerebral palsy may include learning difficulties, psychological problems, sensory defects, compulsive and behavioral disorders of organic origin.

Cerebral palsy as such, then, is not a single disease but a condition characterized by a group of symptoms. It is not a disease that can be described by its cause or etiology. In diagnosing cerebral palsy it is necessary to describe the defects present; to include the parts of the body affected, the extent of involvement, the state of spasticity or flaccidity of the major muscle groups of the body; and to describe any problems associated with hearing, intelligence, vision, speech, or learning.

Historically, cerebral palsy was described in 1861 by William John Little in London. The condition was later called Little's disease, and since that time has received numerous names. The medical profession ultimately accepted the concept of cerebral palsy as a complex disorder of multiple causes and of multiple severities. The term cerebral palsy was coined by Winthrop Phelps, an orthopedic surgeon and a pioneer in the work with cerebral palsy.

The extent of the disease is described by terms that connote the extent of body involvement. Hemiplegia connotes involvement of both limbs on one side. Paraplegia means that there is involvement of both legs with relative or complete sparing of the arms. Quadriplegia means there is involvement of all four extremities. Monoplegia means that only one limb is affected; while triplegia means that three limbs are affected.

TYPES OF CEREBRAL PALSY

Cerebral palsy may also be classified by the types of neuromuscular involvement occurring, using the terms spasticity, athetosis, ataxia, rigidity, or flaccidity. The spastic and athetoid groups combined account for approximately 75% to 80% of the cases of cerebral palsy.

Spastic cerebral palsy accounts for 40% to 50% of the total group, though in many cases it is difficult to isolate a pure form as many spastics seem to have some athetoid movements as well. Typically, spastics have increased muscular tone with a tendency to develop muscle contractures. Children with spasticity usually exhibit exaggerated responses of either flexion or extension and have difficulty combining elements of both. Balance is difficult, and instead of smooth movement their gait becomes awkward and in many cases requires an extended or swinging arm for balance or control. The gait becomes discoordinated, awkward, and they will frequently walk with the toes turning in and knees and hips flexed resulting in a "scissors gait" with toe walking. Because the basic defect involves damage to the motor cortex of the brain, certain muscle groups might be entirely nonfunctional; these muscle groups then are underdeveloped. In the most extreme severe cases, the child is totally unable to sit, stand, or walk and in many cases to even hold his head erect. These children may require special braces and chairs to hold them erect so that any muscles that are still functional may be used to the best capability.

Athetoid cerebral palsy comprises the second largest group, accounting for about 20% of the cerebral palsy population. This type of palsy is due to damage to the basal ganglia in the center of the brain. Damage in this area results in slow, writhing, involuntary muscle activity, characterized by an uncontrolled twisting. This type of movement is called athetosis.

The head and upper trunk and arms are usually more affected than the legs in children with athetosis. They frequently have severe difficulty with head control, with the head being drawn back and twisted to one side. The mouth might be open, and they have trouble controlling salivation. These children walk with a lurching, stumbling, discoordinated walk. They do not pattern well nor follow any particular sequence. Conscious attempts to create movement increase their uncontrolled muscular activity. These children while asleep do not have any jerking physical movements or activity.

Ataxia occurs in about 10% of the cases of cerebral palsy and results from involvement of the cerebellum or its pathways. This part of the brain, located in the back of the cranial vault, is principally responsible for balance. Ataxic children are extremely unsteady and sometimes completely unable to walk. They often have difficulty with eye coordination and have an imbalance of the muscles of the eyes, causing a strabismus or a squint.

A large percentage of cerebral palsied children in our experience have mixed forms, showing spasticity and rigidity and some athetotic movements as well. Mixed forms of athetosis and spasticity are quite common. Less common are mixtures of ataxia and athetosis.

The incidence of cerebral palsy has remained fairly constant through the years and still seems to be approximately one to two per 1000 or 0.1% to 0.2% of live births. This probably does not include all the children with very mild defects as these require no extensive care and are not included in general reporting. Incidence seems to be fairly constant throughout the world. It is unknown at this time as to whether intensive care in prenatal nurseries is going to decrease the incidence of cerebral palsy or perhaps save some children with mild cerebral palsy who otherwise would have succumbed.

CAUSES OF CEREBRAL PALSY

Causes of cerebral palsy are many, and may come about by factors operating at any time during the development of the child.

Infection by rubella or German measles may occur in the infant before he is born. Or the palsy can be caused by maldevelopment or abnormal development of the central nervous system. Trauma or injury is an unusual cause, because the baby is well protected in his water sac in the uterus, but it is conceivable some damage could be caused on rare occasions.

Prenatal anoxia, a premature separation of the placenta, shock, threatened abortion, anemias, or carbon monoxide poisoning can all cause a deficiency of oxygen delivery to the fetus. Certain metabolic diseases in the mother, particularly diabetes, can cause central nervous system damage in the unborn infant.

Rh incompatibility, where there is sensitization of the mother, can cause damage to the brain in two ways. The mother develops antibodies that can attack and destroy the red blood cells in the baby. Because of the rapid breakdown in red blood cells, the infant might have an insufficient amount of blood to supply the central nervous system with the needed oxygen. Or the hemoglobin from the red blood cells that are destroyed may be incompletely metabolized by the liver, with a buildup in the bloodstream of bilirubin. Bilirubin is normally excreted through the bile ducts into the intestinal tract, but if the breakdown occurs too rapidly and the liver is unable to metabolize all the breakdown products, the excessively high bilirubin levels can cause direct damage to certain centers in the brain.

In normal newborns without any blood incompatility, there is a rapid breakdown in red blood cells with the development of what is called a "physiologic jaundice" which can occur on the second or third day of life. The amount of bilirubin in this case does not reach critical levels and does not cause damage to the brain. When there is damage to the brain due to excessively high bilirubin levels, a disease entity called kernicterus occurs. Kernicterus usually results in a severely retarded child in both motor and intellectual spheres.

RhoGAM, a special type of gamma globulin, is now used to prevent the development of sensitivities occurring in women having blood incompatibilities with their infants. Since the introduction of the use of this special gamma globulin, kernicterus has become an extremely rare disease.

More recently, alcohol excess and excessive smoking have both been implicated as being responsible for some types of damage to the unborn child. (See the section on these problems in Chapter 8.)

Injuries during delivery   During delivery there are many injuries which can occur to the infant: difficulties with the placenta, the cord being wrapped around the infant's neck, a knot in the cord, or the cord prolapsing or coming out ahead of the baby, can all cause a decrease in the oxygen supply with resultant central nervous system damage. Breech deliveries, high forceps deliveries, and other abnormal presentations all are responsible for damage on occasion. Recently, more frequent caesarean sections coupled with fetal monitoring during the labor have reduced the incidence of this type of complication.

Prematurity is a frequent cause of cerebral palsy.

Childhood diseases, particularly those infections causing meningitis or encephalitis, cause a high rate of damage to the child's central nervous system. Influenza, mumps, and measles are all responsible for a limited, but significant, percentage of cases. Another frequent cause of difficulty is a head injury caused by accidents in automobiles, in the home, and on the playground. More frequently diagnosed these days are head injuries caused by child abuse which can lead to significant central nervous system damage.

Poisonings caused by toxic chemicals, lead, and carbon monoxide are all capable of causing central nervous system damage and resultant cerebral palsy in infants.

It is estimated that about 10% of cerebral palsies are caused by postnatal insults to the central nervous system.

Multiple pregnancy is also a factor in that twins or triplets seem to have an increased incidence of cerebral palsy. Whether this is due to prematurity or whether it is due to poor oxygenation and poor nutrition because of the multiple pregnancy, is not known.

COMPLICATIONS

Associated with cerebral palsy are other handicaps which, though not related directly to the motor system, do occur because of insult and damage to other important centers within the brain.

Mental retardation is probably the most frequent complication noted beside the neuromuscular difficulties. Investigations indicate that anywhere from 35% to 58% of children with cerebral palsy will have an IQ below 70. Figures coming from Denmark indicate that between one-third and one-quarter of cerebral palsy children are of average to above average intelligence while the remainder suffer from a mild or severe form of mental retardation. Because of the rather bizarre neuromuscular movements and spastic athetoid gaits, at many times there is an unwarranted impression that these children are all retarded. This is not correct.

Visual defects are common in the cerebral palsied child. Approximately 50% of these children will have difficulty with oculomotor movements (the ability to move the eyes together and focus on a specific point). One quarter of this group will have subnormal vision as well.

Hearing loss   Approximately 20% of the children will have a hearing loss of a minor to major degree. It was once felt that this incidence was considerably higher, but careful surveys have indicated that in the athetoid group only 20% to 25% will have hearing loss and only 7% to 10% of spastics show any significant hearing deficit.

Speech defects   Over 30% to 90% of the children will have speech defects of a minor or major degree. Again, pure spastics appear to have less difficulty than the athetoids or those with an ataxic type of cerebral palsy. These are principally articulation difficulties due to poor motor control or delayed speech due to mental retardation and delayed maturation. In certain cases there is a frank aphasia probably due to damage to the speech center in the brain.

Epilepsy is another frequent occurrence in children with cerebral palsy. Surveys indicate that as little as 10% and as high as 50% of the children with cerebral palsy are afflicted with some form of epilepsy. Epilepsy occurring in children with cerebral palsy is no different than that occurring in any other group of children. But our experience has been that, in many cases, these are more difficult to control and require careful supervision of their medication programs.

SYMPTOMS

In looking for early evidence of cerebral palsy, there are four cardinal signs:

1. An abnormal, floppy muscular tone,

158

2. slow motor development,
3. a persistence or continuation of the more primitive neurologic reflexes,
4. unusual or abnormal patterns of motor development.

Developmental guidelines discussed in Chapters 1 and 2 follow a fairly normal progression. If this normal progression is absent or markedly delayed or if there is a continuation of an excessive startle or other primitive reflexes, this is a clue or at least a suggestion that the child might have some damage to his central nervous system.

B.F. Andrews and his colleagues name several items that might be considered red flags.*

The baby has trouble sucking.
He pushes the nipple and food out of his mouth.
The mother complains:
   "I can't get his legs apart to change his diapers."
   "My baby is so nervous."
   "He never moves himself."
   "He cries whenever I pick him up or turn him over."
   "He's slow."
   "He crawls like a bunny."
   "He runs with one arm up."
   "He rolls over too early in life."
The development of definite right- or left-handedness early in life.

Children are usually ambidextrous until 18 months of age or later. If a child consistently prefers to use one hand, he should be suspected of having a motor deficit of the opposite extremity.

None of the items in the list is diagnostic of itself. If, however, one or more of the items is constant enough to create concern about cerebral palsy, this should be discussed with a health professional.

TREATMENT

Treatment programs today begin early in infancy at the time of diagnosis and may continue through adolescence into adult life. Infant intervention programs directed toward the motor and sensory spheres are started early in life. These activities are designed to normalize, insofar as possible, motor activity and to stimulate mental and sensory experiences.

---

*Andrews, B.F., Banks, H., and Blumenthal, E.M. Cerebral palsy: my baby is slow. *Patient Care* January 30, 1979, 1–8.

These activities also provide an arena of discussion for the parents with professionals of several disciplines which might include not only the physician, but also nurses, physical therapists, occupational therapists, speech therapists, and educational specialists.

Preventive care is an active program in the treatment of cerebral palsy children today. In past years, an attitude of "tincture of time" was the prescription frequently given. This resulted, on many occasions, in a perpetuation or even accentuation of the disability. Today, the basic philosophy of intervention is an attempt to achieve as near normalcy as possible, using the child's strengths as well as his weaknesses. All sensory-motor capabilities are developed to their fullest potential.

An active effort is made to prevent contractures and other deformities from developing, particularly in the severe spastics whose flexion contractures of the limbs can prevent any possible usage of that limb at later dates. An effort is made to encourage and normalize the appropriate proprioceptive, tactile, visual, and hearing sensations to the fullest extent. There is also an active effort to minimize the overcompensation of motor activities which leads to posturing and nonfunctional gaits and movements.

An evaluation is accomplished of the deviations from normal in the child's movement patterns. Attempts are then made to utilize other activities to correct these deficiencies as far as is possible.

In treating spastics, the reduction of the spastic muscle tone is paramount to a therapeutic regimen. This is accomplished by specific exercise and activities that tend to relax and break up the muscle spasm.

In the treatment of the athetotic child, the primary aim is to minimize the involuntary movements as far as possible. It is important that these programs be started early in life before the movements become habitual. By minimizing the stimulation presented to the child, purposeless activity can be reduced. Complex activities are difficult and activities in the treatment program must be simple and usually unidirectional. A relatively calm surrounding will reduce some of the reflexive activities by avoiding distracting stimulation.

Ataxic children have severe difficulty with their stability. The treatment program is aimed at developing control in moving the body without losing control of muscle function. These children have marked difficulties with fine motor activity. Its development must progress gradually from gross to fine movements.

Treatment programs must be designed individually for the child depending upon his basic neuromuscular and sensory losses. Treatment must begin early and must continue as long as is necessary to bring the child to his full neuromuscular capabilities. Special equipment, wheelchairs, crutches, bracing might be needed if damage is of that severity. It is possible to develop special eating utensils and arm or leg braces to solve specific problems.

It is important for the parent at home to stimulate the child in all spheres of hearing, sight, sound, as well as in the motor sphere. This requires a vast effort. A program can be outlined, developed, and presented to a parent, but it is only the parent with his minute-to-minute association with the child who can bring the program to fruition.

Parents of children with cerebral palsy must remember that these children will also have their routine share of infections, colds, broken bones, and other medical problems of childhood. It is important that they receive their routine immunizations and that their physical condition be monitored by health professionals.

Hearing should be checked early. If the child has a hearing loss, it should be adequately evaluated and if possible treated or assisted by a hearing aid if required.

Dental problems are frequent in children with cerebral palsy, and careful dental hygiene is important.

Parents of these children should keep careful records of the growth and development of their child, his activities, and when he reaches the milestones discussed in Chapters 1 and 2.

Psychologic complications with cerebral palsy are many, and they affect all members of the family as well as the child himself. Parents, brothers, and sisters frequently need help, understanding, and even counseling to understand the complex problems and the whys of this disease. The child himself as he grows older might require some help and counseling in comprehending his disease and the restrictions that it has placed upon him.

Help of this nature can be obtained from the United Cerebral Palsy Association (Appendix 2), or local mental health clinics. Or referral can be made by local physicians. It is important to seek help early before the worries and concerns become deep-seated and the problems deep-rooted.

14 Epilepsy

Epilepsy is one of the oldest illnesses known and recorded in the history of man, with references occurring in the most ancient medical history. It still remains one of the least understood of common disorders. It is a disorder characterized during medical history as being in the realm of mystery, fantasy, and at times associated with witchcraft.

The broad term epilepsy is used to define a group of disorders characterized by convulsive muscular seizures with or without disturbances in consciousness. It is a chronic condition in which seizures of cerebral origin recur with or without known organic cause. These seizures are associated with disturbances of the electrical activity of the brain. These usually can be determined by an electroencephalogram (EEG) as either a localized or generalized electric disturbance involving both sides of the brain.

In organic or secondary epilepsy, seizures are associated with known organic brain pathology, that is, with brain tumors or where injury or surgery causes damage to the brain with resultant scarring.

The vast majority of epilepsy cases are called idiopathic, meaning "of unknown cause" because no brain damage can be found by present diagnostic techniques. This is not to say that there might not be organic pathology. However, our ability to diagnose minute areas of damage or scarring still remains limited.

Historically, the term seizure is somewhat of a misnomer, as it dates back to a time when it was felt that the victims had been supernaturally "seized" or possessed by demons or devils. Many famous perons in history probably had epilepsy or at least the form of epilepsy that we call a grand mal seizure. These include such people as Saul of the Hebrews, Buddha, Alexander the Great, even Julius Caesar. Jonathan Swift writes descriptions of his disturbances which are suggestive of a form of epilepsy.

Peter the Great had multiple disorders of the nervous system. Historical reports state that he was "always shaking his head and grimacing, and his right arm was never still." Napoleon was reported to have a seizure-type episode on occasion and probably suffered from grand mal-type seizures.

Handel, Shelley, Alfred Nobel, Byron, Dostoevsky, and Vincent van Gogh all suffered authenticated attacks of epilepsy; although the exact form of the disorder differed.

Evidence of Byron's epilepsy is in the following lines:

The sky spun like a mighty wheel.
I saw the trees like drunkards reel,
And a light flashed spring o'er my eyes,
Which saw no farther. He who dies
Can die no more than I died.

(MD, 1975)

In ancient Greece, a person having a grand mal seizure, falling to the ground unconscious, foaming at the mouth with jerky movements of his extremities was assumed to have been seized by a god or demon and was respected for his "sacred disease."

Hippocrates, in his discourse *The Sacred Disease* (400 B.C.), described several different forms of epilepsy, and he concludes:

It is thus with the disease called sacred: It appears to me to be no-wise more divine, nor more sacred than other diseases. It has a natural cause from which it originates like other afflictions. Men regard its nature and cause as divine for ignorance and wonder because it is not at all like other diseases.

During the seventeenth and eighteenth centuries, masturbation and sexual excess were regarded by most physicians as the primary cause of "fits"; castration was frequently advised and in the nineteenth century became the treatment of choice for this disease. Charles Edouard Brown-Sequard pointed out in his exhaustive book on surgery for epileptics that they also employed such treatments as cauterization of the limbs and skull as they believed that these types of seizures were due to disorders of the nervous system. Certain types of seizures cause only one limb to be affected, so in ancient times they even went so far as to advise amputation of a limb.

The misconception that sexual overactivity could lead to epilepsy accidentally produced the first success in chemotherapy of seizure disorders. At this time potassium bromide, which was used to repress excessive sexual drives, was used in the treatment. Bromides, a form of sedative, met with some success in the reduction of seizures, and this remained a standard medication for epilepsy in spite of many unfavorable side effects.

It was not until 1912 when phenobarbital was introduced that a specific drug became available for treating epileptic seizures. This drug proved to be more effective without the serious side effects of addiction occurring with the bromides.

Epilepsy involves people of all ages, though it is more common in children, and many children do tend to "outgrow their seizures." It occurs in all races, sociocultural enivornments, and all walks of life. The chances are good that in the course of walking through the grocery store or down the street one passes several epileptics. They will not be recognized as having this disease unless they happen to have a seizure at that moment.

Epilepsy is still one of the least known and most misunderstood of all medical disorders. Many times people have been misdiagnosed as having a heart attack or of being drunk. The misdiagnosis in many cases leads to unfortunate social recriminations.

The brain is a complex network of nerve cells that transmit impluses from one cell to the other by chemical-electrical impulses. In the course of everyday life the brain shows normal patterns of electrical activity, even while we sleep. These can be determined by an electro-encephalograph or EEG.

The EEG is an instrument that picks up the brain's electrical activity and registers it on a moving strip of paper as a wavy line. Normal patterns of EEGs have been established for many years, and any abnormal patterns can be seen and diagnosed by a professional trained to read these tests.

The examination is accomplished by attaching small metal disks, called electrodes, to the patient's scalp, usually with a sticky tape. They are placed in specific locations on the scalp and simultaneous readings are taken from all the electrodes. During the recording the patient is usually asked to lie quietly, sometimes will be encouraged to go to sleep when a "sleep tracing" is needed. An adult patient or older child will frequently be asked to hyperventilate, or breathe very rapidly, as this can cause some abnormal activity in the brain.

In most cases, small children are sedated with chloral hydrate or some other sleeping medication to help them rest and permit an accurate test to be performed.

EEGs are not always satisfactorily diagnostic of the problem. They can locate evidence of a generalized abnormal discharge from the brain or they can pinpoint localized damage which produces abnormal waves in only one or two electrodes.

WHY DO SEIZURES OCCUR?

In epilepsy there is a temporary buildup of an excessive electrical charge in some, if not a large number, of nerve cells. Under this excessive activity the brain loses control over the body and a number of things can occur. There may or may not be a loss of consciousness. If there is a loss of consciousness, it might be only a few seconds, or it might last for some minutes. There might be some abnormal or unusual muscle activity with contraction and extension of various muscle groups. There can be a loss of memory or conscious thought. There might also be abnormal sensations of the various sense organs such as smell or vision.

Normally during periods between epileptic attacks, the affected parts of the brain work normally, and the person can function properly in his social environment.

There have been many attempts to develop a diagnostic classification of epilepsies. Two classifications are in general use. The terms familiar to most people include grand mal, petit mal, psychomotor, or "Jacksonian" seizures. A more detailed international medical classification of epileptic seizures has recently been proposed to allow a better classification of many types of disease that do not fit into a simple grand mal or petit mal classification. In essence, this scheme segregates the seizures into partial seizures, generalized seizures, unilateral seizures, and an unclassified category. Readers interested in the detailed classification of seizures are referred to Appendix 3 on suggested readings.

Major motor or grand mal epilepsy causes seizures that take the form of blackouts or loss of consciousness with violent shaking of the entire body in patterns of alternating contraction and relaxation (clonic) or of continuous tension (tonic). These are often accompanied by irregular or a temporary short cessation of breathing, drooling, involuntary urination, and a total loss of memory for what occurred during the seizure. Some patients experience a warning called an "aura" of unusual visual lights, sounds, odors, or just an unexplained fear or knowledge that they are going to have another seizure. The patient will frequently have a postseizure "fugue," in which he may feel confused and tired; he may then sleep for a short to long period of time.

Petit mal or absence seizures are usually very short episodes. They usually consist of simple staring, occasionally accompanied by clonic or automatic movements. These staring spells are sometimes mistaken for daydreaming. They may occur with rapid blinking of the eyes or small twitching movements of hands, arms, or face. They usually last only a few seconds and may occur as often as 100 times a day. Following petit mal seizures, the patient usually resumes activity as if nothing happened and does not know that anything has occurred during this time.

Many parents and teachers can be totally unaware that a child is having occasional petit mal episodes and will describe the episode as an apparent loss of attention for a short period of time. One mother came to us complaining that her son was a behavioral problem, as he was "just ignoring me." Closer evaluation by professionals questioned the presence of a petit mal seizure. This was confirmed by EEG; the child has lost his behavior problem and is now paying attention, cured by being placed on medication.

Psychomotor seizures occur with variable manifestations. The most common are mannerisms consisting of staring, smacking the lips, chewing movements, mumbled or bizarre speech, buzzing or ringing in the ears, dizziness. In many cases these are accompanied by bizarre motor and psychic performances—grunting, loud speech, sometimes quite vulgar. Sometimes the patient cannot remember what has happened during the attack. This type of seizure arises from an irritable spot in the temporal lobe of the brain, and in most cases is extremely difficult to treat. New medications and recent treatment utilizing surgical techniques offer increased promise for the future.

Myoclonic seizures can occur both in infants and in older children. When occurring in infants, they are usually extremely severe. These seizures consist of spasms causing massive muscular contractions when the child is lying down. When sitting, the head drops forward, and the child bends at the waist in a "salaam" type of seizure. These particular seizures are extremely difficult to treat and must be followed very carefully by the pediatric neurologist.

About 4% of all children have febrile seizures at one time or another. They usually occur during the first two to three years of life and appear to be directly caused by the rapidly elevating high temperature. About 6% of children having repetitious febrile seizures will develop true epilepsy. Thus the incidence of the disease occurring in children with a history of febrile seizures is higher than in the general population. Whether febrile seizures constitute the beginning of epilepsy or are a cause of epilepsy is still unknown.

In treating a child with recurrent febrile seizures, a physician will direct that the child be given his phenobarbital or other medication prior to the time of onset of the fever. This, of course, in many cases is difficult, as the onset of any illness is frequently heralded by a sudden rise in the child's temperature above normal levels, and a febrile seizure is sometimes the first sign of acute illness. In cases where preventive therapy is advised and is instigated, this treatment must be prolonged, and continuous therapy should be given during the first few years of life.

Breath-holding frequently occurs in childhood. Often, however, this is mistaken for an epileptic seizure. The age of occurrence of breath-holding spells is usually six months to three years and occurs when the child is startled, hurt, scolded, or has some self-induced frustration. He may start to cry, holding his breath in the expiratory phase; he becomes cyanotic, or blue, about his lips and fingers, and can fall limply to the floor. Usually when he falls and loses consciousness, shallow respirations will return; he may have some clonic jerking or rigidity which probably represents a convulsive response to the lack of oxygen. He may appear somewhat confused or drowsy for a short time. Prognosis in these cases is excellent for normal development providing there are no other neurodevelopmental abnormalities.

The prevalence of epilepsy is extensive. Epilepsy affects more Americans than cancer, tuberculosis, cerebral palsy, muscular dystrophy, and multiple sclerosis combined. The Epilepsy Foundation of America estimates that about 4 million people in the United States, amounting to 2% of the population, have some form of epilepsy. These estimates might be low as epilepsy is not a reportable disease.

An estimation by Epilepsy Foundation of America of cost of epilepsy to the United States is approximately $4.4 billion per year. This includes massive costs for aid, vocational rehabilitation, social security benefits, medical care both in the public and private sectors, and unemployment compensation. At the present time, $5 to $10 million is being spent annually in research trying to find better treatment modalities, to develop new and useful drugs, and to set up other rehabilitation programs for the prevention of epilepsy. Epilepsy exceeds all the estimated annual costs of other neurologic diseases combined and is approached only by mental retardation as a public expense.

DIAGNOSIS AND TREATMENT

The diagnosis of epilepsy involves a multipronged approach. It is necessary to have a careful and complete history, physical and neurologic examination, and many times to include x-rays and other specific neurologic studies such as electroencephalograms, computerized axial tomography (CAT) scans, or brain scans done with radioactive substances. Sometimes a spinal or lumbar tap to examine spinal fluid is necessary to arrive at a definitive diagnosis.

Computerized axial tomography is a new radiographic technique that permits us to look at differences in density of tissues inside the skull. Brain tumors, areas of scarring, or other changes in the brain can be diagnosed in many cases using this technique.

Anticonvulsant drugs   The principal modality of therapy for all the epilepsies consists primarily of the use of anticonvulsant drugs. It is estimated that over 50% of the people with epilepsy can have their seizures well controlled with medication and lead full, active lives. The other 50% are difficult to control and must be carefully followed by their physicians. Medication dosages must frequently be adjusted, and different medications must be tried. The vast majority of people under comprehensive medication therapy will require more than one drug to accomplish good control with a minimal amount of side effects.

All the seizure medications are central nervous system sedatives, and as such create side effects, particularly those of sedation. The ideal drug program controls the patient's seizure activity without creating excessive side effects.

It is imperative that parents understand that in the process of developing a drug therapy program, trial and error is necessary to find the right drug and the right amount to render the child seizure-free. Recent techniques permitting accurate chemical determinations of the levels of medication used to treat seizures in the patient's blood have been developed and are making it far easier to develop the correct dosage schedule.

The commonly used anticonvulsant drugs in the United States today are listed here:

phenobarbital (Luminal)	diazepam (Valium)
primidone (Mysoline)	clonazepam (Clonopin)
mephobarbital (Mebarol)	carbamazepine (Tegretal)
diphenylhydantoin (Dilantin)	valproic acid (Depakene)
ethosuximide (Zarontin)	ACTH gel (Acthar)
trimethadione (Tridione)	prednisone

At the present time there is an active search for new compounds capable of controlling difficult seizures. There was a 15-year dearth in the search for new chemical compounds, as it was felt that most seizures were well controlled with drugs then available. Careful evaluation showed, however, that 25% were poorly controlled and another 25% were only partially controlled, with only 50% actually being well controlled. A research project is currently underway at the University of Utah School of Pharmacy evaluating new drugs with anticonvulsion potential. It is hoped that better medications with fewer side effects will become available in the future.

Surgery as a form of therapy is indicated in only a few cases, particuarly those with temporal epilepsy or people who have an organic basis for their disorder. In certain cases where injured areas can be reached by surgical techniques and removed without creating further scarring, this might become the treatment of choice.

Preventive therapy   There has also been a resurgence of interest in preventive therapy in treating patients with a history of a severe head injury in an effort to prevent the first seizure following trauma. This may be quite effective in certain well-defined instances.

There is also more impetus in encouraging physicians to practice preventive prophylaxis for infantile febrile convulsions associated with a high fever. The final data as to usefulness of these programs are still not available, but preliminary work indicates that in cases of recurrent febrile seizures prevention will probably prove to be an important form of therapy.

In the treatment of childhood epilepsy, perhaps the major difficulty is the refusal of the patient to take or the parents to give adequate medication. When given intially, drugs frequently will cause sleepiness, drowsiness, and other side effects which might be alarming to the parents. These should be discussed with the physician ordering the medication, and his advice as to therapy should be followed carefully. The majority of times drowsiness will disappear after a period of time and permit the child to function correctly.

Some patients do not absorb medication well and may need two to three times the usual dose before they reach a point where their seizures are controlled. When patients are taking more than one medication, if a toxic reaction occurs, determining the amounts of each medication in the blood will help to determine which one of the drugs has reached a harmful, toxic level.

The emotional adjustment which must occur with epilepsy is extremely important. A child or an adult with epilepsy should be able to lead a full and normal life. Fatigue, emotional upset, stress, and premenstrual tension are known to increase the frequency of seizures.

The attitude and approach to people with epilepsy has been tremendously modified, particularly during the past two decades. There still remain, however, some restrictive and discriminatory practices in legislation. There is still discrimination in employment, education, insurance, and recreation throughout this country. Most states require proof of a specified seizure-free period before issuing a driver's license, and people with epilepsy are excluded from the military. This is primarily because there is always a concern that a person may have a seizure while driving in the middle of a busy freeway, and military assignments might involve locations where medical care is not readily available. Many epileptics find that they have major problems in securing and holding jobs and obtaining life insurance. Much remains to be done to correct these social attitudes.

Most children whose epilepsy is controlled can and do attend regular schools without difficulties. There are a few special schools designed for the treatment of the epileptic whose control is difficult or not obtainable and who will not fit into a regular school program. Unfortunately, most schools dealing with special education programs are not directed toward the epileptic with normal intelligence but are concerned primarily with the mentally retarded.

Extensive research is progressing into many major unresolved medical questions concerning epilepsy. The current concerns as to what triggers the abnormal electrical discharge and what happens chemically within the brain during a seizure are still to be unraveled. The exact mechanism by which anticonvulsant drugs work, what chemical effect they have on the nerve cells of the brain or on the chemical neurotransmitters are all under investigation; these mysteries still remain to be solved.

PUBLIC EDUCATION

Educational programs are being developed to help the general public understand more about epilepsy and what to do when they see a person having a seizure.

Although petit mal is a very common type of seizure, it is short-lived and no care is required. On the other hand, grand mal and psychomotor seizures appear to be catastrophic. People seeing a person with this type of seizure are fearful, particularly if they are unaware of the cause and have not seen seizures in the past.

The majority of people suffering grand mal seizures do not require special assistance. The seizures generally only last for a short time and will run their normal course. When an epileptic has a seizure in a public place, a call frequently goes out for police or paramedical help. Usually the seizure has ended by the time help can arrive and the epileptic is caused increased embarrassment.

The following *First Aid for Epilepsy* is published by the Epilepsy Foundation of America and outlines what should and should not be done for a person having a seizure.

Keep calm when a major seizure occurs. You cannot stop a seizure once it has started. Do not restrain the patient or try to revive him.

Clear the area around him of hard, sharp, or hot objects which could injure him. Place a pillow or rolled-up coat under his head.

Do not force anything between the teeth. If his mouth is open, you might place a soft object like a handkerchief between his side teeth. (Do not put your fingers in his mouth—he might bite you severely.)

Turn the patient's head to the side and make sure his breathing is not obstructed. Loosen necktie and tight clothing but do not interfere with his movements.

Do not be concerned if the patient seems to stop breathing momentarily.

Do be concerned if he seems to pass from one seizure into another without gaining consciousness. This is rare but requires a doctor's help.

Carefully observe the patient's actions during the seizure for a full medical report later. When the seizure is over, let the patient rest if he wishes.

The only type of seizure that requires emergency medical treatment is a condition called "status epilepticus." In this condition the person goes from one grand mal seizure into another without ever regaining consciousness. This may last for hours and requires hospitalization and care by a competent physician.

It is important to remember that epileptic seizures cannot be stopped and need not be stopped until they run their normal course.

It is important to realize that all seizures may not be indicative of true epilepsy. Toxic agents and high temperatures might cause convulsions, particularly in very young children. It is also not uncommon to see someone who faints for some other reason have a short seizure-type of episode. This probably represents a lack of sufficient oxygen to the brain caused by the faint. It is usually short-lived and does not constitute a true seizure.

ETIOLOGY

Perhaps the most difficult question arising in the doctor's office is, "Why does my child have epilepsy?"

At the present time there is no known answer as to why brain cells suddenly discharge abnormally creating the flurry of electrical activity in the brain which causes a seizure. Scientists working in the field all agree that epilepsy can result from birth defects in the brain due to abnormal development caused by a wide variety of insults. Infections in the mother while carrying the infant, intoxications from uncontrolled diabetes, toxemia in pregnancy, lead poisoning, and other drug insults have all been known to cause seizure problems. General maldevelopment of the brain from unknown causes can result in seizures. Brain injury before, during, and after birth; accidental injuries to the head; chemical intoxications or poisonings after birth; abnormal nutrition; childhood fevers; infectious diseases causing encephalitis or meningitis; brain tumors can all be implicated in certain specific cases. Sometimes, however, an exact cause cannot be found.

Early in the newborn period, hypoglycemia, or low blood sugar can cause neonatal seizures that must be treated actively to prevent severe brain damage. Low blood calcium may have the same effect. Efficient newborn nurseries are preventing most of this type of complication and, where needed, intensive care nurseries are available in most parts of the country.

The role of genetic transmission of epilepsy has undergone considerable debate in the last 15 to 20 years. There has been evidence of some genetic transmission. The idiopathic generalized seizure disorders (grand mal) are more prone to heritable transmission than the symptomatic focal seizure disorders. The recurrence risk that a parent with a genetic form of epilepsy may have a child with a seizure disorder is about one in 15 to 20. In many cases no symptomatic epilepsy occurs, but some abnormal EEGs can be identified in offspring of parents having a known generalized seizure disorder. Because the chances of the disorder in offspring vary with the nature of epilepsy in the parents, it is necessary to establish a precise diagnosis before genetic advice can be given. Competent genetic counseling of parents or of teenagers contemplating marriage and parenthood is important to help them understand the risks associated with having children. These risks are minimal but must be discussed on an individual basis.

PREVENTION

Some preventive measures can lead to a significant reduction in the incidence of this disease.

Good medical supervision during pregnancy and delivery cannot be emphasized too much. Anoxia, trauma, or injury to the newborn infant can cause seizure disorders. The incidence of seizures is higher among premature infants and those infants delivering in a breech or other abnormal presentation, compared to children presenting in a more normal position. New techniques in obstetrics including fetal monitoring and, where indicated, more frequent caesarean sections probably will reduce the incidence of brain damage and resultant seizure disorders.

Acquired metabolic errors of a biochemical nature can occur in the infant due to hypoglycemia (low blood sugar), hypocalcemia (low calcium levels), or vitamin B_6 deficiency (pyridoxine). All these can be controlled by careful testing, diagnosis, and treatment in the newborn period.

A frequent concern arises in women having epilepsy as they contemplate pregnancy. Between 0.3% and 0.5% of all pregnancies occur in mothers who have epilepsy. These women do have an increased susceptibility to seizures through the pregnancy and a tendency toward folic acid deficiency anemia. Sometimes there are bleeding disorders in the newborn child which are probably related to medication. Malformations and neurologic defects are increased in the offspring, and there is concern for genetic transmission of certain types of epilepsy.

Increased susceptibility to seizures can usually be reduced by controlling the woman's disease before the pregnancy and maintaining her on proper, adequate doses of medication through her pregnancy. Careful prenatal care by her obstetrician and neurologist will prevent most cases of increased seizures.

Many of the medications used in treating epilepsy are known to interfere with folic acid metabolism, and this becomes more acute during pregnancy. The use of folic acid must be determined on an individual basis depending on the blood levels or the appearance of any signs of folic acid anemias. The routine use of folic acid has been known to increase seizures in some cases.

Drugs can also cause slow clotting with platelet decreases in the newborn child. This can usually be controlled by the administration of vitamin K to the mother and to the newborn at birth.

Malformations occurring in the babies born to epileptic mothers on drug therapy appear to be a very real thing. The facts are: an infant born to a mother with epilepsy has two to four times the chance of having malformations or neurologic deficits as those born in the nonepileptic population. Whether all these deficits are related to the medication or whether they are caused by lack of oxygen during a seizure early in pregnancy is unknown at this time. Recent studies indicate that anywhere from 70% to 94% of offspring of epileptic mothers will be entirely normal. It is advised that all mothers maintain their medication at normal levels, consulting with their neurologists throughout pregnancy. Perhaps the most severe damage that can occur to the baby is anoxia due to a convulsion in the mother.

In 1975, reports were published identifying a cluster of minor and major malformations called the fetal hydantoin (Dilantin) syndrome. These include cleft palate, harelip, and heart defects as the major defects. The incidence of occurrence is about 2%. Development defects consist of a short nose, low nasal bridge, mild widening of the distance between the eyes, and minor changes in the hands. Mild to moderate growth deficiency and mental deficiencies are said to occur.

Other anticonvulsant drugs have also been implicated and trimethadione (Tridione) apparently has the most serious malformation frequency. It is reported that about 80% of offspring of a mother receiving this drug have some difficulties.

Diphenylhydantoin (Dilantin) was one of the first agents suspected of causing malformation. Phenobarbital has also been suspected in France, but data have not confirmed this in the United States.

Diazepam (Valium) remains an unknown entity at this time. Conflicting reports have been published.

Valproic acid or sodium valproate (Depakene) is reported to be teratogenic, or capable of causing malformations in animals. At the present time, it is not recommended as a treatment for epilepsy during pregnancy.

To date ethosuximide (Zarontin) has not been implicated as a potentially malforming agent. This is an effective drug in petit mal seizures; perhaps it could be used in place of the more dangerous medications.

Many questions as to why these malformation risks were not identified much earlier have frequently been asked. The low incidence is probably the major reason for not identifying these significant malformations, as they occur in a small and widely scattered population. Even today, the association remains partly theoretical and prospective studies are currently underway to develop proper identification.

TRAUMATIC EPILEPSY

Epileptic seizures may occur immediately after a head injury or accident or may occur many months or years after such trauma. The development of seizures depends on the severity and extent of the wound; penetrating wounds are more apt to produce seizures. If the sight, touch, or smell senses are affected, or if infections occur, the probability o. epilepsy is greater. Following an accident, if a person remains unconscious for long periods of time, he is also at greater risk for the development of a seizure disorder.

Prevention of brain damage can be accomplished by the proper use of seat and safety belts in automobile accidents. Driver education as a tool in preventing traffic accidents and padded dashboards and protective mechanisms in automobiles today all help to prevent serious head damage with resultant seizure disorders.

The same can be said for the prevention of head trauma at work, school, and play. Hard hats in construction areas prevent head damage from falling objects. The development of properly fitting football helmets has prevented brain damage in contact sports. Safety headgear for other sports—baseball, soccer, lacrosse—is all-important in the prevention of brain damage.

Intoxications or poisonings can cause brain damage with resultant seizure disorders. Lead is probably the most frequent metallic poison that can lead to epileptic seizures. Infants and youngsters are most susceptible to ingestion of lead paint and lead oxide fumes. Lead-base paints on ceramics, cribs, and interior woodwork is a common source of the poison; the colored ink in comic strips can also contain lead. Ingestion of toxic quantities of lead can induce mental retardation and behavior disorders, as well as seizures. The majority of paints used today within the home do not contain lead, but in older homes it is still common.

PSYCHOSOCIAL PROBLEMS OF EPILEPTIC CHILDREN

Psychosocial problems are quite common in epileptic patients and their families. The most serious hazard of an epileptic disorder may not be the seizure per se but the associated emotional disturbances that can occur in a youngster and in his parents.

Behavior disorders are common in school children, and academic underachievement is frequent. Whether this represents an actual problem in learning caused by the epilepsy or the medication is unknown. It may be that teachers and peers expect a poor showing by epileptics and this creates a cultural problem. Studies are being done in this area, and perhaps better information will be available in the ensuing years.

Disturbed parental attitudes might be a factor in creating some of these psychosocial problems, and in many cases counseling is indicated in helping to alleviate these problems.

There is some evidence to indicate that the medication might be responsible for part of the academic underachievement, and it is important that medications be properly monitored and maintained at their lowest possible dosage.

Academic underachievement can also occur in children having frequent petit mal, or absence seizures, as the frequency of these can interfere with the thought processes. The child basically receives his scholastic input with many blanks occurring in the teaching environment. It is quite easy to see that if a child is having 20 to 50 petit mal seizures per day and actually loses conscious contact with the teaching instruction, the input to him will be very fragmentary and chaotic. In this case, proper medication will help to increase the academic achievement.

Behavior problems frequently occur, particularly in teenagers and adolescents. Many of these children are worried about "being different," and they have great concern about having a seizure in class and being pointed out as an abnormal person. Relationships with peers as a concern starts quite early in elementary school and continues throughout the years of schoolwork.

The types of problems appear to change as the child matures. Where teasing and social isolation were common in elementary school, the teenager's peers are more accepting of the illness and its symptoms. The child with epilepsy now fits in the group better and appears to be the same and not a different type of child. This has become increasingly true during the past one to two decades.

There still remain many major areas of restriction for teenagers with epilepsy, particularly in the areas of athletic activities. Restrictions in social life appear to be minimal, although many parents are unwilling to have their teenagers stay overnight with a friend, because they are afraid the child will have a seizure and be embarrassed. (A very similar thing occurs in children with bedwetting.) Certain athletic endeavors are restricted either by well-intentioned or perhaps unknowledgeable parents or coaches. They range from not being allowed to swim to curtailment of skating, bicycle riding, regular gym classes, football, baseball—all types of athletic endeavors.

In most cases of epilepsy it is not necessary to restrict any activities providing there is reasonable monitoring. A child with uncontrolled seizures should certainly not be allowed to swim alone or to ride motorcycles, bicycles, or use other types of hazardous transportation in areas of congestion where he might damage himself or someone else. Children with epilepsy due to brain damage caused by accidental injury perhaps should not participate in contact sports. However, these are decisions that must be made individually and in consultation with the physician.

It must be emphasized that many schools are afraid of sick children, especially those with epilepsy. This is primarily a problem of increasing knowledge and developing better communication with the school authorities and teachers concerning the patient's problem and treatment program. An education program for school authorities and teachers is quite important. Programs that have been presented by the author to teachers are well received; indeed the teachers request more information about epilepsy.

Parents of a child with epilepsy should involve themselves in a careful education program, both as the student and teacher, to understand better the cause and treatment of seizure disorders, both medically and psychosocially.

Informational pamphlets on prevention, medical and social management, research, and a bibliography of reading materials on epilepsy are available from the Epilepsy Foundation of America. Their address is listed in Appendix 2.

15 Learning and Behavior Disorders—A Mixed Bag

It becomes necessary to combine a discussion of learning and attentional disorders with behavior disabilities, as they are tightly intertwined in these children's difficulties. Most children seen with one of these problems are found to have an element of another as well. These children are probably the most perplexing and frustrating of all, for parents, teachers, and physicians. The child by his disruptiveness threatens the classroom and the home; he can present with a group of symptoms that can be polygenic, global, or limited, and in many instances difficult to diagnose. For this reason, such a child usually requires a multidisciplinary approach to diagnosis and therapy.

Confusion surrounding these disorders is reflected in the variety of labels. Over 70 different suggested titles and labels have been reported in the literature; they run the gamut from minimal brain dysfunction (MBD), hyperactive impulse disorder, learning disabilities (LD), hyperactivity, hyperkinesis, organic learning and behavior disorders, and the most recent label, attention deficit disorder (ADD), to mention only a few. The terms MBD, LD, and ADD are used interchangeably in this chapter. Many researchers might disagree with this form of "lumping together," but it is felt by the authors that the concept of this disability can be better understood if these classifications are combined.

Because of the input from various disciplines, particularly medicine, psychology, and education, multimodal approaches have been used in attempting to define, distinguish, and treat these disorders.

It is the authors' opinion that these disorders represent a syndrome complex, having not one single cause but multiple causes. The children may present many symptoms that have a wide range of expression.

This disorder affects approximately 5% of school children, though it has been reported to occur with an incidence as high as 20% in some studies. It is characterized by multiple difficulties consisting of patterns of abnormal behavior, attentional or perceptual deficits, excessive purposeless hyperactivity, and difficulties with social and emotional interactions. The child may show an impaired ability to concentrate and to finish tasks. If these are coupled with perceptual deficits, he has difficulty with learning and is labeled "learning-disabled" (LD).

This disorder has been estimated to occur predominantly in boys, from five to nine boys to each girl reported. Certainly the more disruptive, conspicuous form of MBD is much more common among boys than girls, though there is some question at this time as to whether some of the attentional deficits shown in young girls might constitute a "silent" form of this disorder.

The predominance seen in males might be caused by a variety of factors. Active, aggressive behavior is accepted as a normal form of masculine behavior, and social pressures restrict this in girls early in development. Recent reports showing functional differences in the male and female brain have been reported, apparently due to the influence of certain hormones during prenatal life.

The ten most common findings in children with MBD/LD/ADD are:

1. hyperactivity
2. short attention span—inattentiveness
3. distractability
4. impulsiveness with aggressive behavior and difficult peer relationships
5. incoordination
6. perceptual impairments
7. disorders of memory and concept formation
8. learning disabilities (reading, arithmetic, writing, spelling)
9. speech and language problems
10. neurologic and EEG abnormalities

To this group must be added other findings which include frequent mood changes, depression, emotional instability, and anhedonia—the inability, or reduced ability, to experience pleasure.

Children with this type of disorder may have one or many of the findings listed above. They may have a pure, simple hyperactivity problem or a pure learning disability problem, etc. Figure 15-1 demonstrates how these might be interrelated to this diagram of just three behavioral traits. It can be seen that the combination of symptomatology can be very complex or very simple.

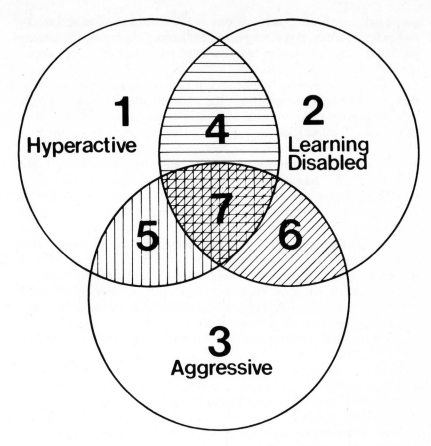

Figure 15-1 Diagram showing mixing of symptoms in the MBD child. (1) Hyperactivity only. (2) Learning-disabled only. (3) Aggressive only. (4) Hyperactive and learning-disabled. (5) Hyperactive and aggressive. (6) Learning-disabled and aggressive. (7) Hyperactive, learning-disabled, and aggressive.

PATTERNS OF HYPERACTIVITY AND BEHAVIOR DISORDERS

Extreme examples are children presenting with severe hyperactivity, showing a total inability to remain on task, coupled with aggression and severe impulsiveness. At the other end of the scale are children with simply a dyslexic problem or a mild hyperactivity without any learning disabilities. It seems incongruous, but there are hyperactive children whose motor activity is less than normal—below that of their classmates. These children may show nothing but an attention deficit with a resultant learning disability.

Hyperactive behavior must be regarded as pathologic when it is accompanied by a short attention span and distractability, when it is purposeless, irrelevant, and not directed toward a specific meaningful task in which the child is supposed to be engaged. The inability to concentrate and perform structured tasks is a hallmark of the hyperactive school-age child.

Historically, many of these children have been hyperactive or exceptionally active since birth. In many cases, mothers have reported that the child was extremely active even in utero with a frequent statement that, "He almost tried to kick his way out." These children frequently have early manifestations of excessive activity. They have feeding problems and do not develop rhythmic patterns of eating and sleeping. Colic and milk allergies are frequent. They are not "cuddly," lovable babies, but want to fuss and squirm all the time. Sleeping difficulties are variable, but most do not go to bed and sleep is erratic. Paul Wender tells of parents giving a history of a child who was active and restless in infancy, stood and walked at an early age, and then "like an infant King Kong burst the bars of his crib asunder and strode forth to destroy the house." (See Appendix 3, Minimal Brain Dysfunction, Wender, Paul H.)

Parents frequently mention that the child is "into everything" and is constantly touching with his hand, inadvertently breaking toys and objects, and having to be watched at all times for his own protection. He has no fear and will try anything. There is frequently a history of the child wandering away from home, having no fear of the consequence of falls, automobiles, or traffic.

Attempts to document a gross increase in motor activity with objective measuring devices have only been variably successful. Some reports show an increase in activity, others no gross increase but only a marked increase in purposeless or useless behavior, accompanied by a high rate of distractability, the child frequently being unable to focus on a given task. Some children give the impression of hyperactivity because of their constant shifting of activities and lack of goal direction. Other children are noted for their inability to inhibit activity when inhibition is appropriate. Excessive motor activity of children with MBD may decrease with age as does the motor activity in all children. Other types of activity and the high distractability rate do not necessarily disappear, however, and may continue into adolescence and adulthood.

Shortness of attention span and poor concentration can be very striking. Parents will report that these children will never play at one game for any long period of time and usually will not sit and watch television programs for prolonged periods. A child will continue to talk while trying to watch a program and wander aimlessly about looking for other things to do. Many times, children are difficult at the dinner table, eating a few bites, wandering around, then coming back to finish their meal.

Cognitively, these children manifest varied patterns of difficulties in learning, particularly in reading and arithmetic skills. Whether the problems of attention span or of cognitive learning deficits contribute more to the MBD child's academic troubles is hard to say, since either would be sufficient to cause difficulties.

Psychologic testing may be totally normal or may show a spotty intellectual deficit with a low normal performance on drawing and block design tests. A large number of the children with MBD will show immaturity in the Bender-Gestalt or the Goodenough Draw-a-Man test.

Underachievement at school is the problem most often precipitating referral for diagnosis and treatment. The problem is compounded by the psychological consequences of early underachievement. A vicious circle results: poor achievement creates criticism, causing a poor self-image, which creates further underachievement and results in a marked decrease in motivation.

There are many changes in the manifestations of this disorder as the child grows. There appear to be some physiologic alterations with maturation, particularly a decrease of motoric hyperactivity. There are also learned psychological alterations—a child is much more hostile after his tenth year of pure rejection than he is after one or two years of such treatment. Problems are socially defined and dependent many times upon cultural expectations. A fidgety, hyperactive nursery school-child is expected and tolerated, while a restless second grader is not. Reading difficulty is expected in the first-grade child, but it is not tolerated in the third grade and is frequently classified as dyslexia in the fourth.

It should be emphasized that not every MBD child progresses through a standard pattern. Some children manifest difficulties in all development stages, some in only a few. Not all children will have difficulties in all areas at any one time. Some will have academic problems; some will have social problems; some will have neither. These children may outgrow not only their hyperactive problems but other difficulties as well, provided they are not permitted to become chronic failures in their school activities. It is usual for these problems to abate at or around the time of puberty.

Studies are just beginning to look at the MBD child-turned-adult. These findings are significant in that many of these young adults are showing significant personality disorders. There is a high incidence of alcoholism in these people as well as other forms of sociopathy. Hysterical antisocial behavior is common in women. This would tend to indicate that the problem is continuous, and though the manifestations diminish and change, some persist either as a result of a basic physiologic biochemical defect or as a result of psychologic and social conditioning that has occurred through the child's life. Older MBD subjects often report continued difficulty in concentration, and many of these individuals manifest an absence of sustained interest in nonacademic areas as well, such as recreational activities, hobbies, and jobs. All these activities initially attract their attention but fail to maintain their interest. It is not unusual to find an adult MBD who is moonlighting on two or three jobs, not always for financial security, but in many cases to satisfy desires or demands for a high activity level.

TREATMENT

The treatment of the child with MBD must be individualized. There must be a careful assessment of the child's defects, level of activity, and a careful evaluation of his intellectual capacity. By definition, a hyperactive child is one of normal intellect. This does not mean that hyperactivity cannot occur in the mentally retarded as well, because it does quite frequently. Treatment in both areas is essentially the same but must be modified for the child with decreased intellect.

It is necessary to have a careful evaluation of the social and cultural backgrounds of the MBD child. It is also necessary to evaluate carefully his educational background and to determine whether he has developed the basic learning skills necessary for reading, writing, and arithmetic.

His psychologic behavior should be carefully evaluated. Are there severe emotional problems in the child or in his family? Are there behavior problems that need to be modified to develop the atmosphere that would permit good learning behavior?

It is obvious that this analysis requires a multidisciplinary approach if success is to be obtained, with interaction between the physician, educator, and psychologist or behavior modifier.

Educational treatment requires careful evaluation of the defects in the basic learning skills the child may have acquired in kindergarten through the second grade. Techniques are now known to educators to ascertain which of these skills are absent, and programs for developing these skills in children can be accomplished.

Perhaps the most important thing the educator and the parent have to accomplish is to see that the child with normal intelligence does not fall drastically behind his peers but is kept up to date and that special approaches are used wherever necessary to accomplish educational goals.

Recent reports using a multidisciplinary approach show that 75% to 85% of hyperactive children are progressing through school and graduating from high school without significant academic deficiencies.

Psychologically, at the time of diagnosis, many of these children have a lot of bad learned behavior that must be modified in some way so that the behavioral difficulties do not compound the distraction. Many techniques for this may be used by both the parents and the educators. On occasions, a specific program of behavior modification is necessary; it must be prescribed for an individual child and must be monitored by a competent psychologist. It is important to remember that many of these children are unable to experience pleasure (anhedonia). This makes it difficult on a reward-and-punishment basis to accomplish behavior modifications, but if these programs are carefully developed and monitored, this can be done.

The medical therapy requires, first of all, a diagnosis. This should include a careful history and physical examination to determine whether there are any frank physical or neurologic deficits. In the vast majority of cases, children with the entity do not demonstrate frank neurologic abnormalities. There may be "soft signs" which suggest some abnormality, but these by themselves are not diagnostic.

The physician should ascertain by history whether there is anything suggestive of a seizure disorder, as there is an increased incidence of such disorders and abnormal electroencephalograms in this population of children. In cases where there is a suggestive history, an electroencephalogram should be done to rule out any problems which require a different form of medication therapy. The general feeling among most neurologists treating this disease is that EEGs are not needed in all cases, but they should be done in specific instances.

Stimulant medication therapy is the hallmark of medical treatment and is effective in approximately 70% to 80% of hyperactive children. (The paradox of "stimulating" the hyperactive will be discussed presently.) It has two major effects on the motor activity of the child: 1) to decrease the hyperactive behavior, and 2) to increase the attention span. It must be emphasized that no one has ever demonstrated that children treated solely with stimulant drugs, without educational and behavioral therapy, subsequently do any better in their long-term education programs than untreated children.

The paradoxical effect of stimulant drugs, that they calm the child rather than stimulate him, appears to be due to the fact that these drugs act on an inhibitory center in the midbrain; when stimulated, the center becomes more active and decreases the excessive motor activity of the child and his distractability. This response to medication would suggest that there probably are some specific biologic differences between hyperactive and normal children, at least in some children. This is currently under extensive investigation.

It is important, if medication is used, that it be carefully monitored by the physician and that it be used in the lowest possible dose to achieve effective results. Dosage might have to be varied as the child grows older and bigger. Frequent contact with the child's physician is imperative. Stimulant medications used to treat children with MBD/ADD are the amphetamines (Dexedrine), methylphenidate (Ritalin), and magnesium pemoline (Cylert). In situations where there is an inadequate response or where there is a problem with depression, the tricyclic antidepressants may be used in treating these children. The principal tricyclics used are imipramine (Tofranil) and amitriptyline (Elavil).

In the majority of cases, the stimulants are tried first as they are easier to regulate, side effects are less troublesome, and they have a relatively short half-life; the drugs are excreted quite rapidly from the body without any accumulation.

It is interesting in treating these children to note that tolerance does not usually develop requiring an increased dosage to maintain effect, nor do there appear to be any addictive difficulties. Medication can be stopped abruptly without creating withdrawal symptoms.

The long-term side effects of stimulant medication appear to be minimal as long as the child is correctly monitored and minimum dosage levels are maintained. There may be a brief retardation in growth which might be due to an induced anorexia from the stimulant medication, but this corrects itself. These children frequently show other signs of delayed maturity compared to their peers; they tend to be less coordinated, more clumsy, and their growth is frequently delayed. This appears to be only a delay (usually about one year), as these children will ultimately reach their anticipated genetic growth.

Because of the multiplicity of behaviors and the probable multiplicity of causes of this entity, various therapies have been introduced in an attempt to treat the learning-disabled or hyperactive child. Various therapeutic trials have been made, but the ultimate efficacy of these remains to be determined by careful clinical investigation.

Bennett Feingold of San Francisco has presented a theory that food additives cause hyperactivity and has reported his results in treating children with a dietary program. Careful evaluation of his diet programs is currently under way.

Megavitamin therapy, the use of large doses of vitamins far beyond those apparently needed in the average person, has also been tried.

Behavior modification programs, special schools, meditation, hypnosis, biofeedback are all techniques that are currently under investigation.

Not all these programs have been adequately subjected to scientific scrutiny, nor have they been supported by the scientific community. Carefully clinical trials still are required before they can be advised as a proper course of therapy.

Questions concerning any of these programs should be discussed with your physician for information as to the current thinking and knowledge of any of these programs. The information is changing rapidly and can have changed drastically from the time of the preparation of this book.

While the vast majority of MBD children will respond to a medication program coupled with educational and psychological intervention, there still remain 10% to 20% of the affected children who are unresponsive. To a certain degree these children, with proper programs, can be trained to develop better work habits, increased attention span, and consciously to control their activity levels. Special training of this type is available only in certain areas of the country in a few of the major research centers.

All parents of hyperactive children should realize that there are some basic things to be avoided. A child with a short attention span should certainly not be expected to sit through a four-hour opera. Because of decreased coordination, distractability, and short attention span, such sports as little league baseball should probably be avoided; the sitting and waiting may not be tolerated. Soccer, and in some cases, football or basketball, where there is rapid activity, can make good activities for these children providing their coordination will permit them to participate adequately.

Parents of hyperactive children should discuss their concerns carefully with the health professional guiding therapy of their child. Perhaps the most common mistake is adopting an attitude of "it will go away." While it is true many of the symptoms will disappear, the basic attentional deficit may remain. The secondary problems that develop in the untreated child are sometimes difficult to correct, for example, serious basic deficits in his three-R skills.

Becoming a chronic and constant failure can lead to an extremely low self-image and severe depression. The pressure exerted by his peers at times can be cruel and harmful. The child becomes known as a "dummy" or a "retard" and frequently develops a reputation among teachers as being a troublemaker—a reputation that can be extremely difficult to live down even if his behavior and academic skills improve markedly.

It is imperative that the child be *reinforced positively* any time that his performance is adequate, and certainly the praise should be profuse when his performance is outstanding. Positive reinforcement can go a long way in ameliorating poor self-concept.

The causes of hyperactivity are still unknown. In searching for an etiology, investigators have tried to pinpoint distinctions between normal and hyperactive children. This has proved to be extremely difficult, probably because the causes are polygenic and multitudinous.

In many investigations, hereditary influences are markedly strong, and it is possible to find reports of hyperactive parents, grandparents, aunts, and uncles. It has been suggested that in these cases perhaps there is a genetic biochemical defect that is transmitted from one generation to another.

It is known that brain damage can also cause symptoms of hyperactivity. One of the early descriptions of hyperactive children was reported in a group of children damaged by a severe postinfluenza encephalitis in 1918 to 1920. Children born to mothers with toxemia of pregnancy and diabetes and children who have had periods of hypoxia, or lack of oxygen during birth all have an increased incidence of hyperactive behavior.

Many hyperactive boys and girls have significantly more minor physical anomalies of certain sorts. Frequently the fathers of these children also have an unusual number of these minor anomalies: slightly malformed or asymmetrical ears and changes in the fingers or toes. None of these physical changes is sufficiently constant to add any help in specific diagnoses.

Investigators are still far from determining the actual causes of this syndrome, probably because there are multiple causes. Until something definite is determined, prevention will be difficult. Treatment at the present time is limited to medication, specific educational programs, and where indicated, specific behavior therapy.

16 Emotional Disorders

Most parents do all they can to promote healthy emotional development in their children. When certain behaviors appear in children, parents often have difficulty recognizing differences between abnormal behaviors and those behaviors that are seen in children exhibiting normal development. The following examples illustrate the complexity of emotional development, and the difficulties parents encounter in knowing whether their child is behaving normally or not.

A mother and her three-year-old child are shopping at the supermarket. The child is continually touching many of the items on the shelf, and the mother can be heard scolding the child repeatedly. The child ignores the mother, goes about his merry way wreaking havoc on the shelves. Is this child emotionally disturbed? A five-year-old sister comes up to her three-year-old younger brother and demands that the brother give her his toy. He refuses. The older sister at this point begins hitting the younger brother. The younger brother cries and refuses to give his toy to his sister. Is either of these children emotionally disturbed? Finally, a three-year-old child refuses to go to any other adult but his mother or father. Is this child emotionally disturbed? The purpose of this chapter is to clarify, and hopefully demystify, popular misconceptions regarding emotional problems in children. Parents who possess accurate information are better able to make sound decisions regarding their child's development.

One of the major concerns of most parents is what is "normal behavior"? A primary notion that is widely accepted in the psychological field is that normalcy is a relative concept. That is to say, that normalcy much like beauty, is in the eye of the beholder. Cultures define beauty; cultures define normalcy. Consequently, we can see that much of what parents decide is normal behavior for children is defined by the culture in which they are raised and whose values and concepts they are taught.

187

Many philosophers and psychologists have argued that there are universal sequences of social and emotional development. However, it is rather clear that child-rearing practices as well as notions about appropriate child behavior, differ from culture to culture and from family to family. One culture may value aggression and assertiveness in their male offspring and may encourage these characteristics. Another culture may prize and value passivity in their male offspring, and in fact train their male children to be passive.

Parents can make distinctions between normal and abnormal behavior by asking two important questions: "Is the child's behavior a problem for the child?" and "Is the child's behavior worrisome or inconvenient to those who interact with the child?" These are mainly his parents, teachers, peers, family, as well as society at large.

CLASSIFICATION

Many attempts have been made to classify emotional disturbances. One of the most widely used classification systems is that published by the American Psychiatric Association. They divide childhood behavior problems into organic or biologic problems, and functional or nonorganic problems. Other classifications have used the same two basic categories.

Research in the area of childhood emotional disturbance suggests that they cluster around two major variables: conduct problems that are related to aggression and "acting out" and personality problems related to anxiety and withdrawal. A third variable might be inadequacy—ie, immaturity. Different investigators have different categories of childhood emotional problems. Indeed, there may be little practical importance for a parent to know the different labels when it comes to doing something about his or her child's problem behavior. While classification of behavioral disorders may provide professionals with a handy method of categorizing them, such an approach does not in and of itself resolve the emotional problems displayed by children.

CAUSES OF EMOTIONAL DISORDERS

Not only do numerous systems for classifying emotional disorders exist, but various investigators in this field have hypothesized different causes of emotional disturbances in children. The idea that a child's behavior problems are caused by one specific factor is a common misconception. Also, it is commonly assumed that each behavior problem takes only one specific form. Actually, it is quite rare that a child's behavior problems are singular in nature or that they are caused by only one factor. For example, a child with behavioral problems may have difficulties that stem from a brain injury or neurologic impairment. In addition, other causes such as emotional stress or the rewarding of inappropriate behaviors may contribute to the problem. Therefore, any statement regarding the cause of a child's problem is more likely to be a description only of the primary cause. There may well be other secondary causes or factors of lesser significance.

Hereditary and Biological Factors

Emotional disturbances, including neuroses and psychoses, have been investigated for years to see if they have any clear genetic bases. Research has shown some weak genetic factors may exist, but no absolute conclusions can be drawn. Future investigations may lead to the discovery that some emotional disorders may well be linked to a genetic cause. For example, research has indicated that childhood schizophrenia may be a metabolic problem. Certain proteins needed for healthy nervous system and brain functions are not properly assimilated by the child's body. The number of behavioral and emotional disorders currently believed to be inherited, however, are few. One possible exception is problems related to mental retardation where strong evidence indicates a genetic cause for many types of retardation. At this point it does seem safe to say that hereditary factors set limits for different capacities, development, and physical stature.

Other physical factors such as intelligence can determine or influence the child's behavior. Physical stature, as mentioned previously, can have a marked effect on the child's type of behavior and adjustment. Physical abnormalities can be very traumatic in the lives of young children. They can cause behavioral and emotional problems because of frustration, unhappiness, and anger. By and large, however, most of the behavior problems seen in young children stem from learning socially unacceptable means for dealing with their environment.

Learned Disorders

Genetic, organic, cultural, and linguistic functions are known to influence the development of emotional disorders. Nevertheless, the majority of behavior problems, particularly the less severe, nonpsychotic problems, are learned. The philosopher John Locke stated that the child's mind at birth resembles a "tabula rasa" or blank slate. Learning follows the interaction between experiences in the environment and the child's biologic boundaries established at conception. But generally, it is believed that the way a child behaves is a function of how he learns to behave.

The environment in which most early learning takes place is the family. Parents and professionals agree that up to at least the age of five, the majority of the influences upon the child's behavior come from the parents. The family may be viewed as a system in which all members are rewarding and punishing one another, as well as sending different types of communications to one another. Children and parents mutually affect each other's actions, and the child's behavior can reinforce certain acts of the parents. Thus, the problem behavior of the child does not result directly from the parents' actions, nor should they be blamed for the child's actions. Take, for example, late night crying. This common situation occurs when a child cries at bedtime, and then asks to be allowed to stay up later and watch television. The parents initially say no, and the child cries harder. So eventually the parents give in, and by doing this they reinforce or reward the child's crying behavior. The child at the same time reinforces the parents, however. They realize that if they allow him to stay up and watch television he will not cry. Since his crying is unpleasant to them, they will allow him to stay up in order to avoid the unpleasant scene. Thus, by stopping his crying only when his parents "give in" he rewards their giving in. This makes it easier next time he wants to stay up because his parents will tend to give in sooner. In general, it is useful to think of the family as an integrated system in which deviant behavior on the part of any member can occur and is maintained through a complex pattern of learned inappropriate responses.

It seems quite clear that learning has a strong influence on the development of emotional disorders. Children act inappropriately because they have learned to do so. These inappropriate behaviors have been rewarded or punished in the past, and the child continues acting in a disturbed manner as a result of this previous learning.

Finally, some emotional problems such as overdependence, poor concentration, restlessness, tempter tantrums, and enuresis (bed-wetting) tend to show a more pronounced decrease with age than do other disorders such as chronic disobedience. Therefore, the social significance of a behavioral problem alters according to the age of the child. Qualitative changes occur with age in a variety of syndromes.

The causes of emotional disorders in children are many. Rarely will one disorder result from a specific cause, such as inadequate parental guidance, faulty learning, genetic predisposition, or cultural determinants. Most often all of these factors interact in a complex fashion and influence the way a child behaves.

FORMS OF EMOTIONAL DISORDERS

Having examined some of the reasons why emotional disorders might occur in children, we now can explore some of the specific forms of disturbance children often display. They can take numerous forms, and the following description covers only the major or general types seen in children.

It is useful to look at conditions in young children considered emotionally disturbed as part of a continuum. At one end are minor behavior problems, and at the other extreme are the psychoses or most severe disturbances. In the middle of the continuum are the so-called psychoneuroses or personality disorders. Such things as enuresis, excessive temper tantrums, and the like, are found in many young children, but they are considered to be of minor importance unless they persist as the child grows older. If they do persist, the child is often called emotionally disturbed.

The psychoses on the other hand, are characterized by highly disturbed thought and behavior patterns. The individual lacks contact with reality to the extent that he or she is unable to function as a normal individual. The specific psychotic conditions of schizophrenia and autism involve a withdrawal from social contact and often evidence a variety of bizarre behaviors.

Fortunately, most of the problems that parents deal with are relatively minor. The process of growing up does not always proceed smoothly, and most children exhibit at one time or another some abnormal behaviors. It is to be expected that various socializing forces including the family, the peer group, the school, and the community modify the adjustment process for each child. Some children will react with excessive aggression, others will become timid and shy, and others will react with frustration and anger.

Aggression

Since a certain amount of aggression is highly rewarded in our society, it is not unusual to see children behaving in overly aggressive ways.

Children subjected to frustrations that are experimentally produced frequently exhibit aggressive responses, particularly if the environment is permissive of this expression. In one study, preschool boys and girls were watched while playing with dolls for two 30-minute sessions. During the first session, they were playing freely. However, before the second session, one group of subjects, the "frustration group," worked on an extremely difficult task that made them feel unsuccessful and frustrated. The control group was not experimentally frustrated before the second play session. In the second session, both groups displayed more aggression than they had during the first play period. This can be attributed to the nonpunishing or permissive atmosphere that permitted such expression. The frustration group, however, showed significantly greater increases in aggression than the control group. Apparently, frustration elicited the subsequent heightened aggressiveness. Not only is the amount of frustration a factor in subsequent aggression, but also we find that some children have a higher tolerance for frustration. We have quite often seen in our treatment center that children with a high frustration tolerance are more successful in the preschool experience. They can tolerate more interference and frustrations imposed by their peers and teachers in the natural give-and-take of life.

Another factor in children's expression of aggressive behavior is the style of upbringing in their homes. Parents who are permissive and allow their children to be more expressive of frustration or aggressive and angry feelings, are more likely to see angry or aggressive outbursts when and if the situation warrants it. Other children who are punished for these types of aggressive behavior, are less likely to evidence appropriate situationally-defined aggression.

Many parents are uncomfortable with children expressing anger, particularly if it is directed at them. Expression of anger can be healthy for children if it is done in a nondestructive fashion, such as verbalizing it. However, hitting other children or breaking household property should not be excused. Parents need to teach their children to be assertive in verbalizing their anger and frustration so they can feel better, but not to damage anyone or anything. Assertiveness is expressing one's likes and dislikes without attacking or belittling another person.

In summary, we see that aggression can be a function not only of the situation but also for the child's history of experiences. If a child is told repeatedly by the important adults in his environment that he is an aggressive child, he will respond to the demands and expectations of these adults by acting aggressively. Similarly, children who have aggressive parents can learn that aggression is an appropriate means of dealing with one's frustrations and problems.

Dependence

Another developmental problem relates to the overly dependent child. Dependency is related to the need for adult approval, affection, and attention. Certainly it is clear that dependency and independence are two ends of one continuum and most children fall somewhere between these extremes. Whether or not a child is "overly dependent" or has "high dependency needs" is a function of age and development. The assertion that a child is overly dependent is a judgment made by the adults in this child's environment. Obviously, a two-year-old should be seen as appropriately dependent on mother and father; however, at this age most children begin to explore their environment and to assert and demonstrate more independence. Typically, children in their fourth and fifth years who manifest the clinging type of dependency we see in children aged two and under can reasonably be judged to be overly dependent. These children quite often have overly protective parents or guardians. These are parents who do not encourage independence, autonomy, and self-reliance, in fact encouraging the opposite: namely, dependency, lack of autonomy, and lack of self-reliance.

Children who are overly dependent are also prone to acquire fears and phobias and be excessively anxious. Although fears and phobias are very common in children, their prolonged presence usually requires some type of intervention. The most common fears are of animals, darkness, and separation from parents.

A specific type of phobia in children that usually requires intervention is school phobia. School phobia is suspected when a child refuses to attend school because he or she is afraid. Fortunately, a variety of treatment approaches are successful in treating it.

Hysterias, Obsessions, and Compulsions

Closely related to the fears and phobias that occur in children is a group of behaviors called variously hysterias, obsessions, and compulsions. Hysteria involves an involuntary loss of motor or sensory functions and in children usually manifests itself in sleepwalking or sudden emotional outbursts. Obsessions typically take the form of thoughts that the child is unable to control. For example, a child may have thoughts about dying that become so persistent and intense that he is unable to control them. Compulsions, on the other hand, are behaviors that are repeated in a ritualistic fashion. It has been suggested that obsessions precede compulsions in children. If a child is obsessed with thoughts about dying, he or she may develop elaborate behavior patterns to guard against these thoughts.

Many parents have heard the expressing "terrible twos," which refers to the fact that at age two, a child begins to refuse to follow some of the parental commands and expresses some temper. It is true that the child's refusals increase during this year, and he objects to routines and commands and resists social pressures. However, severe tantrums are not characteristic of age two. Many professionals counsel parents to accept the oppositional behavior of the two-year-old as a healthy sign of self-awareness and an assertion of budding individuality. It is at this time that the child learns to be more self-reliant and somewhat independent. The child who is resistant can simply be prompted through a task by physically taking him through it, if necessary, and playing down or ignoring the verbal refusals.

Temper tantrums, however, can often grow out of proportion during this two-year-old phase. Let's take a closer look at how tantrums develop. The goal of tantrums is the parent's reaction. The child wants the parent to give in. When a parent allows the child to get his way, tantrum behavior is reinforced, and the possibility of its future occurrence is increased. Tantrums can be dealt with much the same way as oppositional behavior. That is, the child can be picked up and taken through the task physically, telling him that he *will* do what mom or dad wants. Another strategy is to ignore the tantrum. "Time out" has also been used in dealing with tantrums. This is essentially banishing the child for a brief period of time to his room. When using this procedure, it may be advisable to take all toys from the room so that there is little attraction for him during this time. Also, the parent should insist on two to three minutes of quiet and not two to three minutes of screaming. It is important to keep in mind that paying off the tantrums (by giving in) will increase them in the future. It is also very important to praise the child for ending the tantrum.

Perhaps one of the more common behavior problems seen in preschool children is sleep disturbances. Sleep is essential to the child's ability to handle frustrations and to perform his activities daily. Furthermore, unresolved battles over sleeping habits can create ill feelings between parents and children. It should be noted, however, that resistance to sleeping and night wandering are common problems in the preschool child. Children, when put in bed, often spend a period of time fussing. If the parents retain anxiety about the child's sleep and continue to pick up the child whenever he fusses, he may become tense, tired, and wakeful.

Children over two years of age, tired or not, are able to postpone sleep for two or three hours after they are put to bed. Young children can cry in pitiful whimpers or indignant screams while older children can repeatedly summon their parents with requests for drinks, conversation, or trips to the bathroom. Quite frequently, we see that children resist bedtime because they do not like to be excluded from parental activities. Having been prevented from joining the adults in the living room, the child manipulates them to visit him or her in the bedroom. Another cause can be that a preschool child varies his sleep because he is afraid of the dark or is worried about his parents leaving him. Often, when children are unprepared for a babysitter and have awakened to find their parents gone and a stranger with them, they have shown a fear of sleeping for many weeks thereafter.

Psychoses

Our discussion of emotional problems would not be complete if we did not further consider the severe emotional disorders known as psychoses. Until the publication in 1941 of Charles Bradley's book on childhood schizophrenia, there was little or no literature to be found on the topic. In the ten-year period from 1946 to 1956, however, 542 titles appeared. This interest is all the more remarkable because psychosis in any form is rare in childhood.

Clinicians have reached the point of agreeing that childhood schizophrenia exists, but the definition is best left a broad one. Thus, schizophrenia is characterized by defective interaction with reality that displays itself in disturbances in emotion, movement, perception, speech, thought, and social interaction. Original behavioral criteria proposed by Bradley and Bowen for diagnosing childhood schizophrenia are the following:

1. seclusiveness
2. irritability when interrupted
3. daydreaming
4. bizarre behavior
5. diminished number of personal interests
6. regressive nature of personal interest
7. physical inactivity
8. sensitivity to comment and criticism

The schizophrenic child might show a variety of atypical behaviors, such as emotional withdrawal or overt dependence, extreme joy and fear, strange mannerisms (finger-waving, self-destructive behavior such as head-banging, and peculiar posture and gait). Other manifestations include disorientation of space and time, muteness, idiosyncratic verbalizations, and loose associations in thinking. We need not look at psychosis as a more extreme case of neurosis or a step further along a neurotic-psychotic continuum. Rather, the severely disturbed child might never go through a phase that could be called normal or even neurotic. Psychotic children are not simply more disturbed; their object relationships are disturbed in very special ways and quite often they do not progress through the normal stages with normal developmental anxieties. Their development proceeds along different lines at different rates.

Autism

It is generally agreed that psychiatrist Leo Kanner first used the label "autistic child" or "autism." In an article, Kanner described 11 children whose behavior patterns during development appeared unique and whose symptoms appeared to constitute a unique syndrome. This was termed "early infantile autism." In his clinical description, Kanner emphasized that the autistic child has not had a withdrawal from established contact with others (ie, a regressive defense), but had always been aloof. So, unlike most psychotic children, these children had never withdrawn from the social environment; rather, they never interacted with it, being "alone from the start."

In 1943, Kanner noted that these children comprised about 10% of all psychotic children, with more boys being affected than girls, as in all psychoses. Autistic children look normal. In fact, they usually seem somewhat bright because of their alert, thoughtful expressions. Their motor coordination seems normal; indeed, they usually move quickly and are energetic and skillful with their fingers. Their pathology is soon evidenced, however, by their avoidance of another's eyes and by a lack of visual or auditory responses to others. In a sense, they appear to be deaf and blind to other people.

Looking back on the early developmental history of these children, one can see that there are early signs of severe problems even in the infancy period. There is typically no evidence of pleasure in the mother's company or evidence of a social smile. Mothers of these children are typically heard to report, "He didn't look at me when I fed him in my arms." Other complaints include, "He was never cuddly," or "He never noticed when I came into or left his room." There is no evidence of any physical reaching out, he does not call out to be lifted up into his parent's arms. In addition, there is no particular fear of strangers that is so common in the first year of life. Often they are regarded as very good babies, mistakenly, because they do not fuss or demand the parent's time.

Thus, we see a child who appears to be self-sufficient and far happier when left by himself. It has been noted that impaired language development, hereditarily determined, might be a contributing cause to the child's extreme withdrawal. The child, unable to rely on his own consistency of responses to given stimuli, is continually startled and maintains his security only by a major reduction in the amount of stimulation to which he must react.

As noted earlier, this syndrome is more predominant in boys. Dr. E.L. Phillips pointed out that autistic children are predominately first-born boys. He hypothesizes that quite frequently, parents find themselves in a dilemma over setting controls and limits for the first child as opposed to permitting freedom of action. This might be more acute in the first-born son. The child becomes increasingly unsure of his ability to assume full responsibility for his action. Yet, he is committed to do so by his parents' ambivalence, and he retreats to the protection of a limited and controllable environment. Current research has tentatively credited this disorder to biology and heredity gone awry. Future research may well link autism to biologic factors.

What is the prognosis or hope for cure for the psychotic child? Dr. Kanner reported that of 96 autistic children, only 11 were found to be caring for themselves in their second or third decades of life. Interestingly enough, several of these attained a college education; some were employed, for example, as truck loading supervisor, accountant, bank teller, and general office worker. They had hobbies; most lived alone. Few had romantic relationships and personal friendships, which appeared not to be frustrating. Dr. Kanner attempted to account for the successes of these former psychotic children, but he was only able to come up with two indicators: all 11 of these people had speech before the age of five years, and none of them had spent their early years in state institutions.

It is generally agreed that the prognosis for childhood psychosis is poor. While there are many different treatment programs currently existing, no one treatment seems to ensure a good outcome. Rather, what we see is that there is a direct relationship between the original severity of the dysfunction and the prognosis—that is to say, the more severe the early childhood pyshosis, the less chance for later adjustment. For this reason, it is important to stress the importance of early intervention in treating various types of emotional problems.

17 Educational Programs for the Handicapped

After finding out that a child is delayed, there are a number of alternatives for parents. In this section we will briefly attempt to discuss some educational possibilities for handicapped children. Before we do that, however, it may be helpful to outline some of the history behind education for the handicapped.

In the past, programs for delayed children have been few and far between. Part of the problem stemmed from the fact that there had been little dialogue between the medical and the educational communities. Too often, physicians were stumped when there was no specific medical or operative procedure they could suggest which would alleviate a child's handicap. Unfortunately, some doctors advised parents to "institutionalize and forget about" even mildly handicapped children early in life when they had no other solution. Consequently, many handicapped children were put into institutions or hidden away at home starting at a very early age, and were never given opportunities to develop normal skills or to prove that they did have potential to learn. On the other hand, members of the educational community were not properly trained to work with handicapped children, especially the severely handicapped. Because school systems were only responsible for the education of children ages five and up, teachers rarely came into contact with handicapped children. We all remember *The Miracle Worker* or similar stories about a dedicated teacher who makes great progress teaching a child so handicapped that all others, including parents and doctors, have given up any hope. But again, these cases were rare, and in reality very few handicapped children were taught in a systematic manner.

Slowly the dialogue between medicine and education has been opening up, and now people are beginning to realize that a concerted effort is necessary in order to provide the best services for delayed children. It seems apparent that educators must become more familiar with medical terms and conditions, while medical personnel must become aware of current educational methods. Universities are now offering courses designed to prepare students majoring in education and in medical specialities to provide services to meet the total needs of the handicapped child. This is a relatively new attitude toward the handicapped, however, and consequently, the quality of services varies greatly in different parts of the United States.

Regarding federal legislation for the educational rights of handicapped children, Public Law 94-142 was passed by Congress on August 23, 1977. This law expanded and revised Part B of the Education of the Handicapped Act. This new law required states and localities to establish priorities for providing a free, appropriate public education to all handicapped children. The first priority was to the most severely handicapped children within each disability who were receiving an inadequate education.

A free appropriate public education is now mandated for all handicapped children between the ages of 5 and 18 within all states, and free public education for all handicapped children between the ages of 3 and 21 is mandated in many states. However, for handicapped children ages 3 to 5 and 18 to 21, this clause was not applied in any state if its application would be inconsistent with that state's law or practice, or with the order of any court with respect to public education within such age groups in the state.

The guidelines for education of the handicapped vary across the country, just as education for normal children varies from state to state. Before the passage of the Education of the Handicapped Act and Public Law 94-142, many handicapped children were receiving no formal education at all. Now, all handicapped children from ages 5 to 18 must be provided with a form of education that meets their individual needs.

The type of education that will be provided for each child not only depends on his handicapping condition but also on the resources available in the school district where he lives. The parents must be willing to work with the local educators to determine what type of available placement is most appropriate for their child. If an appropriate educational setting is not available in the area, it is the state's responsibility to pay for the child to be educated in the nearest appropriate school.

A discussion of the different types of educational alternatives available may be useful. Most school districts have special education teachers for all grade levels. These teachers have specialized training to work with children who are learning-disabled, emotionally handicapped, or mentally retarded. If the child's handicapping condition in one of these areas is not too severe, he is most often admitted to the local public school and placed in either a self-contained classroom for handicapped children or in a resource room. A self-contained classroom is usually one in which a small group of children with various handicaps spend the day working on specialized programs, either individually or in small groups. A resource room is a classroom to which a child will go for part of the day to receive specialized help in the academic areas in which he has difficulty. Throughout the remainder of the day the child attends a regular classroom with normal children his own age.

The current trend is to encourage parents and teachers to allow the child to be "mainstreamed" into the regular classroom as frequently as possible. The concept of mainstreaming handicapped children refers to integrating handicapped children into normal school programs. It is felt that the handicapped child benefits from social interaction with normal children and from the enriched educational environment, while the normal children benefit by learning to interact with handicapped people early in life.

In most areas, local schools are not staffed adequately to educate blind or deaf children. These children are most often placed in schools dealing specifically with these handicapping conditions. At these special schools the blind or deaf child is taught how to function with his handicap in addition to learning academic skills. These schools are most often residential centers where the child stays throughout the week for comprehensive 24-hour-a-day training.

Education for the physically handicapped child will vary with the degree of his disability. If the child is only moderately disabled, he can often attend the local schools. As the severity of his disability increases, however, the more difficult it may be for him to receive services. Architectural barriers are often the main features that keep a child out of a normal school. A building with many stairs and no elevator or with a bathroom door that is too narrow may bar a normally intelligent but physical handicapped child. Many new buildings, both public and private, are being designed to be barrier-free as public awareness of the problem grows. It is important that the child be placed in an educational setting that provides physical therapy as well as emphasis on academics.

Often a child's handicap is too severe to be dealt with even if the family and the local schools work together. State homes or institutions exist in every state and provide alternatives to the schools already mentioned. These vary from state to state; however, most state institutions have begun to modernize their services and facilities. Children who are placed in a state institution are usually quite handicapped, and the decision for placement is arrived at only after careful consideration by the child's family and doctors.

The important thing to remember is that there are alternatives for the education of handicapped children. With parents and educators working together, every handicapped child can have an educational program to fit his needs.

INFANT STIMULATION

Although legislation will eventually provide therapy for the education of all handicapped children, the child from birth to age three has been neglected in many areas of the country. As studies have shown, this age group is the one that can benefit most from an early intervention program. This now brings us to what services are available and where to look for them.

Although many professionals do not like the term "infant stimulation," it does convey the general meaning. Infant stimulation refers to presenting appropriate development skills to a child from birth to age three in a consistent manner. This can be done in a variety of ways and by a variety of people. Here is a brief description of what each one does.

A speech pathologist, or speech therapist, works with children who are deficient in their ability to communicate verbally. This ability is generally divided into skills involving both speech and language. Speech implies that ability to produce sounds correctly, while language implies the ability to convey meaning through correct word usage and sentence structure. A child who has difficulty making the sound "s" or "l" has a speech problem, while a child five years old who speaks only one- and two-word phrases has a language problem. Some of the disorders which necessitate the help of a speech pathologist include articulation problems, stuttering, vocal modules, mental retardation, and cleft palate.

An audiologist specializes in testing for hearing difficulties and then prescribes hearing aids for the child when necessary. An educational audiologist has a background in speech pathology as well as audiology. This kind of therapist works with the hard of hearing, teaching them to communicate through lip reading, sign language, or a combination of both.

A physical therapist, specializing in physical disabilities, works with children to teach them to use their muscles. Some of the disabilities generally treated by a physical therapist working with children include cerebral palsy, brain damage, spina bifida, juvenile arthritic diseases, amputations, cystic fibrosis, as well as many others. Therapy may vary from teaching a child with only one leg to use an artificial limb, to providing a cerebral palsied child with the basic movement patterns necessary for normal rolling, sitting, standing, and walking.

An occupational therapist has a similar education background to that of a physical therapist but specializes in teaching activities of daily living to handicapped children. This includes teaching feeding, dressing, and other self-care skills. Another major area of expertise of the occupational therapist is developing the function of the arms and hands.

CHILD HELP PROGRAMS

State, federal, and private sources have funded programs to demonstrate the effects of early education for handicapped children. After a child has been identified as having a development problem, several different types of programs may be available to the parents.

A center-based program in which the child is treated by professional therapists is probably the most traditional approach and the most expensive. In this method the parents usually bring their child to a hospital or child center for evaluation. Depending on the philosophy and availability of staff members, the child would receive periodic treatment from one or more therapists. The frequency of the therapy visits might vary from several times per week to once a year. The cost of the evaluation and the therapy visits is generally left to the parents and can be quite expensive. There are some programs, however, that charge for treatment on a sliding scale based on the size of the family and income. The advantage of this form of treatment is that the child is treated by professionals and if seen often enough may show good gains in development. This type of care is generally available only in larger communities, is very expensive, and is quite limited in the number of children that can be seen on a daily basis.

A center-based group program is another method of serving handicapped children. Parents bring their children and meet in a group conducted by a teacher or therapist. The children are evaluated by a team of professionals before they enter the program. The program is designed so that the therapist is the overseer of the children, but the parents are the ones who actually work with them. This type of program may be conducted daily or at least two or three times a week. The parents' availability and participation are required with this form of program. The charges for a "center-based group program" may vary from no fee to a moderate charge for services.

A home-based program is a third model for serving handicapped children. A professional or an aide visits the home and conducts the therapy sessions. The person visiting the home may be a public health nurse, a therapist, or an aide who is trained to conduct home visits and work with delayed children. The child usually has been seen by a doctor or team of professionals before participating in this type of program. The professional or aide might visit the home on a weekly, bimonthly, or monthly basis and perform therapy with the child. Depending on the philosophy of the program, the therapist may also leave a list of some activities or exercises for the parent to do with the child. Many of these programs are federally- or state-funded and are available at little or no cost to the family. They can be effective especially in rural areas because the family does not necessarily need to live close to the program and usually many children who live distances apart can be served.

These are only three general ways in which handicapped children receive services in the first years of life. They may not be available in all communities. It seems, however, that if parents become more involved with a child's early care and development, it is more likely that the child will eventually attain his greatest potential in life.

Here are a few suggestions to parents on becoming more involved:

1. Become an authority on the child's problem. Read as much as possible about his problems and include the whole family in learning about them.

2. Do not be intimidated by health professionals. They should not talk down to you. Being knowledgeable about one's child and his problems is the best safeguard against this.

3. A parent should know his and his child's rights by keeping up with current legislation and being willing to get involved with organizations for the handicapped.

4. Be willing to work with the child. So many parents let teachers do all the work. Waiting until a child is in school before he gets any stimulation or instruction loses precious time.

5. Be proud of the child's accomplishments, and do not dwell on his shortcomings. Although your next-door-neighbors may "feel sorry" for parents or children, they can learn to see the child as an individual by pointing out his accomplishments, no matter how small they seem.

6. Treat the child as normally as possible and discipline him as you would your other children. Too often parents are afraid to discipline their handicapped child and as a result, many of these children become spoiled.

18 What Does the Future Hold?

What are the hopes and the dreams for the next decades? What are the promises on the horizon for help for the developmentally disabled?

George Tarjan, a pioneer in the field of mental retardation and the Director of the Mental Retardation and Child Psychiatry Division at the Neuropsychiatric Institute of U.C.L.A., had these things to say at the Harry A. Waisman Memorial Inaugural Lecture on October 26, 1977:

Amniocentesis and fetal diagnosis are small steps forward. Not too far from now, we'll be doing fetal surgery for repairing damage that cannot be repaired after the immune system has matured.

Fetal monitoring will produce knowledge that will enable women to select ideal pregnancy times and ideal labor times. We already have knowledge that allows us to distinguish mature fetuses from immature ones by looking at lung maturity. A better understanding of the onset of labor might enable us to postpone labor until maturity occurs.

We know enough now to provide most newborns with an intact nervous system and with an environment that is supportive of intellectual, emotional, and social growth.

The most important developments that lie within our grasp concern the modification of genetic disorders. Look at PKU: the treated individual with PKU bears little resemblance to the untreated infant. New breakthroughs like this one lie just around the corner.

How much more would we know about mental retardation if we understood the meaning of competence, not of incompetence?

How much more could we do for the retarded individual if we had as good a scale to identify his strengths as we have now to identify his shortcomings?

How much more could we do about assessing our early intervention programs if we had normative data about impaired younsters' normal growth and develolpment?

How much more could we do if we knew more about language development and development of communications among retarded people and between retarded individuals and others in their environment?

The most important contributions will probably not come from the identification of additional single disease conditions or errors in chromosomes or metabolism, but from a better understanding of the process that leads from those errors to mental retardation.

I also expect within 10 to 20 years revolutionary treatment changes such as minifilters for the removal of toxic substances and organ cell implantations for the treatment of certain conditions.

Most important is research in the biochemistry of the developing fetus. The implications in this area are great. We already have made amniocentesis possible. An open arena follows.

The great hope for the future appears to lie within three separate arenas and, much like a three-ring circus, activity goes on in all rings at the same time. Also like the circus, there is a ring-master who maintains order, permitting the activities in all three arenas to flow from one into the other.

In the first arena is the prevention parade. From this ring will emerge better understanding of genetic mechanisms, better and more knowledgeable counselors with better diagnostic techniques at their disposal. This will not become a "eugenic" society, where people will be told when, how, and where to breed, but it will permit people to make better and more rational decisions concerning their children.

A few areas of genetic research have only just been touched, and perhaps someday in the not-too-distant future, it will be possible to replace or change abnormal or missing biochemical systems within the human body.

David Smith, a dysmorphologist at the University of Washington, Seattle, pleads that the concept of total motherhood begins prior to conception and continues throughout the child's lifetime. We will learn better how to avoid the insults to the developing embryo and fetus. We will learn better how to treat the mother and her diseases so as to prevent damage to her unborn child. Better treatment of illness, accidents, and injuries to the child during and after birth will prevent many of the disabilities seen today.

In the second arena is the treatment animal. More specific treatment will become available for specific diseases. True, we will not be able to remove the extra chromosome from a Down child, but perhaps we can invade and at least partially negate the biochemical effects that this extra chromosome creates. Hearing loss and blindness may someday respond to the whip of the electronic "trainer," permitting us to stimulate those centers of the brain responsible for the interpretation of these senses. Better and safer medications will be forthcoming to treat people with seizure disorders, diabetes, infections, and other errors of metabolism.

In the third arena are the acrobats—the hit of the show. They are those dedicated people who work hard at their art of teaching, for these are the educators. Educators of special children must be two-thirds teacher and one-third actor if they are to develop the teaching techniques that will reach these handicapped children. They must at times be sad, stern, and forceful;

at other times, they must be happy and able to dance and sing as they teach their young charges. Special education programs are progressing and will develop into better programs designed more specifically for each individual child's handicaps, for every child must be brought to the full upper limits of his capabilities, be they great or be they small.

And the ringmaster, coordinating, supporting, and keeping order, is the parents helping their child receive the best possible education.

This is what we foresee for the future. It will require work, investigation, research, and the dedication of a multitude of people working with developmentally disabled children.

19 Using the Personal Health Record

The Personal Health Record chart is included here to assist parents in collecting information regarding their child and his growth and development (Figure 19-1).

Information concerning how to measure the child and record the information is given. Any abnormalities noted—illnesses, seizures, and a short history of illnesses in blood relatives—should all be written into the chart. Any special tests or examinations should be recorded when they are done, as should the child's immunizations. If space is insufficient, any notes can be continued on the back side of the record.

Information on this record, or the record itself, can serve as a great source of information to any health professional evaluating the child.

Figures 19-2 through 19-5 are charts that were compiled by the National Center for Health Statistics in collaboration with the Center for Disease Control of the U.S. Department of Health, Education, and Welfare. They are based on data from national samples representative of boys and girls in the general United States population. They can be used to direct attention toward any unusual body measurement. Even though it can be normal in any given individual, it might indicate some evidence of disease or poor nutrition in another.

HOW TO USE THESE FIGURES

Measuring the child   All infants and children up to 36 months of age should be measured nude or with minimal clothing and without shoes. Until the child is able to stand erect, the length can be measured with the child lying on his back fully extended. Two people may be required to measure a child properly; one person holds the child's head and the other marks the length at the heels. Older children may be measured standing erect, recording their height against a flat surface such as a wall or door.

In measuring weight, ideally a beam balance should be used in preference to bathroom scales, which tend to be inaccurate and to vary frequently. The children should be weighed with minimal clothing or nude up to age 36 months and after that time with minimal indoor clothing or underwear. Future weight measurements should have the child wearing essentially the same amount of clothing.

In measuring the child's head circumference, the measurement must be made at the largest circumference—from the forehead to the back of the head.

Recording   After all measurements are taken and recorded, find the child's age on the horizontal scale, then follow the vertical line from that point to the specific measurement (length, weight, or head circumference). Where these two lines intersect, make a mark with a pencil. When the child is measured again, the marks may be joined by a straight line.

Interpretation   Each figure contains a series of three curved lines numbered to show selected percentiles. These refer to the rank in a group of 100. When a cross mark is on the 95th percentile, it means that only five children among 100 of a corresponding age and sex had measurements greater than that recorded. Conversely, a mark on the 5th percentile means that only five of the children show lower measurements and 95 have greater measurements.

Any child showing measurements consistently in the 95th percentile or above or the 5th percentile and below should be evaluated carefully by a physician. Children should also be evaluated by a trained professional if there is any consistent, rapid increase in any measurements, eg, a sudden and persistent change from the 50th to 95th percentile.

A flat or decreasing measurement curve also warrants careful evaluation. The occurrence of these types of abnormalities does not mean that a disease or a severe abnormality is present, but they do require careful evaluation.

PERSONAL HEALTH RECORD

Name_____ Birth Date_____ Parents_____

Date of Measurement	Age	Length	Weight	Head Circumference	
	Birth				

Development

Sat up_____   Vision_____
Crawled_____   Hearing Loss_____
Walked_____   Allergies_____
Simple Words_____   _____

Congenital Abnormalities _____
_____

Seizures

Type_____
Frequency_____
Medication _____

Is there a history of any of the following among the blood relatives?

Diabetes_____   Genetic Disorder_____   Type_____
High blood pressure _____   Congenital Abnormalities _____ Type_____
Epilepsy _____   Cancer_____   Type_____
Developmental disability _____   Type_____
Other_____

PATIENT IMMUNIZATION RECORD

Recommended Ages and Actual Dates of Administration for each Antigen

DTP		POLIO		MEASLES	
Ages	Date	Ages	Date	Age	Date
2 mos.		2 mos.		15 mos.	
4 mos.		4 mos.			
6 mos.		6 mos. (opt)			
18 mos.		18 mos.			
Boosters:		Boosters:			
(4-6 Yrs.)		(4-6 Yrs.)			

RUBELLA		MUMPS		OTHER	
Age	Date	Age	Date	Age	Date
15 mos.		15 mos.			

Special Tests and Examinations:

X-Ray: When_____ Where_____ Results_____ Physician_____

EEG: When_____ Where_____ Results_____ Physician_____

EKG: When_____ Where_____ Results_____ Physician_____

Brain
Scan: When_____ Where_____ Results_____ Physician_____

Special
Lab: When_____ Where_____ Results_____ Physician_____

Injury or Accident _____ When_____ Where_____

Hospitalization or Operation _____ When_____ Where_____

Illnesses _____ When_____
    Continue on back of page if needed.

Figure 19-1 A child's personal health record.

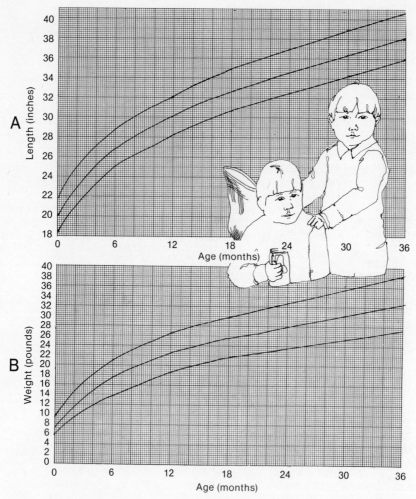

Figure 19-2 **A** shows boy's length from birth to 36 months with the 5th (lower curve), 50th (middle), and 95th (upper) percentiles indicated. **B** shows boy's weight from birth to 36 months with same percentiles. **C** shows boy's head circumference from birth to 36 months with same percentiles.

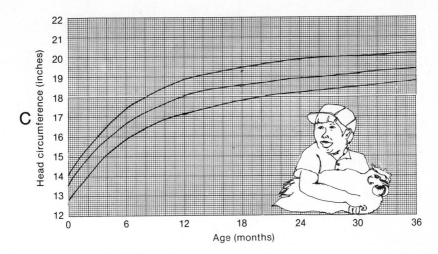

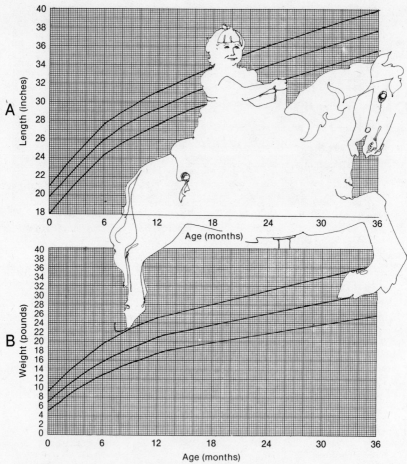

Figure 19-3 A shows girl's length from birth to 36 months with the 5th (lower curve), 50th (middle), and 95th (upper) percentiles indicated. **B** shows girl's weight from birth to 36 months with same percentiles. **C** shows girl's head circumference from birth to 36 months with same percentiles.

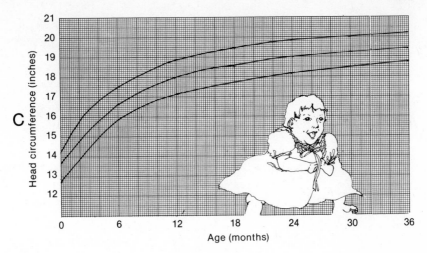

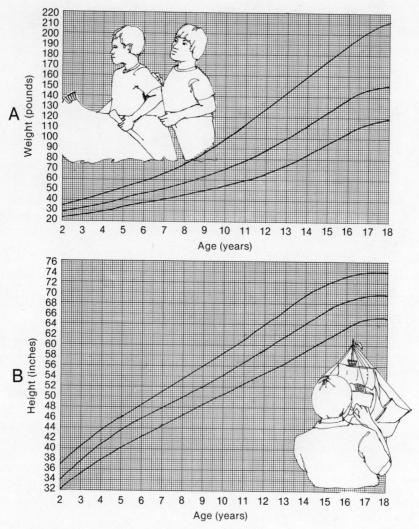

Figure 19-4 **A** shows boy's weight from 2 to 18 years with the 5th (lower curve), 50th (middle), and 95th (upper) percentiles indicated. **B** shows boy's height from 2 to 18 years with same percentiles.

217

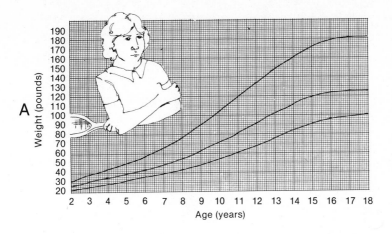

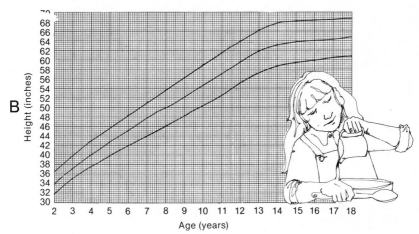

Figure 19-5 **A** shows girl's weight from 2 to 18 years with the 5th (lower curve), 50th (middle), and 95th (upper) percentiles indicated. **B** shows girl's height from 2 to 18 years with same percentiles.

GLOSSARY

Achondroplasia A hereditary, congenital deficiency of bone formation resulting in a type of dwarfism.

Adenoma Glandlike skin-tissue tumor, usually benign.

Alleles Two or more contrasting or alternative forms of genes occupying an identical site (locus) on sister homologous chromosomes. Alleles determine alternative inheritance characters (for example, light or dark pigmentation).

Amaurotic Pertaining to blindness without any apparent eye lesion.

Aminoacidopathies Inborn errors of metabolism which affect amino acids, or protein substrates.

Amniocentesis A procedure for diagnosing genetic abnormalities in utero. Amniotic fluid is taken from a pregnant woman. Chemical contents of the fluid are studied directly for the diagnosis of some diseases. Cells are cultured, and metaphase chromosomes are studied for detection of chromosomal irregularities (eg, Down syndrome).

Amnion The inner fluid-filled sac in which the embryo develops in higher vertebrates.

Amniotic fluid Liquid contents of the amniotic sac of higher vertebrates containing cells with the chromosomal content of the embryo (not that of the mother). Both fluid and cells are used for diagnosis of genetic abnormalities of the embryo or fetus.

Anemia Abnormal condition characterized by pallor, weakness, and breathlessness, resulting from a deficiency of hemoglobin or a reduced number of erythrocytes.

Aneuploidy Deviations from the normal diploid complement of chromosomes, eg, 45-hypodiploid, 47-hyperdiploid.

Anomaly That which is markedly irregular, exceptional, or deviating from typical, not necessarily diseased.

Anoxia Lack of oxygen.

Aphasia Loss or impairment of ability to use language due to brain damage.

Athetosis Abnormal, involuntary occurrence of slow, writhing motions of the extremities, particularly the upper extremities.

Atonic   Without tone. In reference to seizures, atonic attacks are episodes of sudden loss of muscle tone or drop attacks.

Atrophy   Wasting away, degeneration, decrease in size.

Aura   The warning symptoms of a seizure. In fact, these are partial sensory symptoms which are stimulated by a local area of abnormal discharges in the brain.

Autosomes   The nonsex chromosomes consisting of chromosomes No. 1 through 22 (22 pairs).

Cafe au lait spots   Flat, tan spots on the skin about the color of creamed coffee; seen in many disorders including neurofibromatosis.

Canthus   A corner or juncture of the eyelids.

Carcinogen   A substance capable of inducing cancer in an organism.

Carrier   An individual which carries a recessive gene that is not expressed (ie, obscured by a dominant allele).

CAT scan. Computerized axial tomogram   A laboratory procedure utilizing x-ray diagnosis where a computer is used to reconstruct the cross sectional densities of tissues by plotting the relative absorption of x-rays. A plot is made which visualizes the deep structures of the body.

Centromere   The primary constriction connecting the strands of mitotic chromosomes and separating the two arms.

Cephalocaudal development   The growth process observed in children in which the child first gains control of his head and upper portions of his body before he can control his legs. The term actually means "head to foot."

Cerebellum   The portion of the brain which controls coordination of movements, located at the top of the spinal cord and at the very base of the brain itself.

Cerebrum   The cerebrum consists of the two major hemispheres of the brain; each of these hemispheres is made up of a frontal, temporal, parietal, and occipital lobe. The cerebrum contains the centers for intelligence, memory, motor control, and sensory preception—speech, vision, language, and so forth.

Chromosome banding   Staining of chromosomes in such a way that light and dark areas occur along the length of the chromosomes. Lateral comparisons identify pairs. Each human chromosome can be identified by its banding pattern.

Chromosomes   Nuclear structures containing DNA, the material which has the genetic information encoded in it.

Chromatid One of the two identical units resulting from self-duplication of the chromosome during division.

Cleft lip, harelip A lip that is congenitally split, or cleft.

Cleft palate A congenital fissure or split down the middle of the palate.

Clonus Rhythmic jerking movements.

Concordance Usually refers to twins and indicates they have the same trait. Discordance is the opposite term.

Congenital Present at birth. Genetic influence not implied.

Consanguinity Refers to mating between blood relatives.

Cryptorchidism Undescended testicles.

Cytogenetics Area of biology concerned with chromosomes and their implications in genetics.

Deletion Loss of a part of a chromosome or gene.

Dermatoglyphics The study of ridge and crease patterns in the hands and feet.

Diploid The double state of chromosomes (and genes) in normal somatic cells (in humans $2n = 46$).

Dizygotic Fraternal twins; identical twins are monozygotic.

Dominant When a single gene of a pair produces the full effect in the presence of a different allele on the sister chromosome. Codominant refers to the situation in which the single gene is expressed but less strongly than if two were present. Incomplete dominant is the same a codominant.

Dominant inheritance Genetically speaking, this refers to gene traits which are expressed in one family generation after another, usually with variations in the degree of their expression.

Electrocardiogram—EKG—ECG A graphic tracing of the electrical current produced by or causing the contractions of heart muscle. It detects irregular rhythms, rate, and diseases causing abnormal electrical conduction patterns.

Electroencephalogram—EEG A technique for recording brain waves or electrical impulses in the cortical or surface brain cells.

Embryo A young organism in the early stages of development; in man, first period in uterus.

Enzyme A protein that accelerates a specific chemical reaction in a living system.

Erythroblastosis Jaundice in the newborn due to incompatibility in blood groups (A, B, O) or Rh.

Eugenics The science of improving the qualities of the human race; the application of the principles of genetics to the improvement of mankind.

Extensor In reference to seizure activity, this indicates the position of the arms and legs in extension such as extensor rigidity or extensor clonus.

Fetoscope An instrument that may be inserted into the uterus of a pregnant woman to detect structural characteristics of the fetus.

Flexor In seizure activity, this term refers to the position of the arms and legs in flexion.

Focal Refers to a selective localization either in reference to distribution in brain waves or distribution in movement patterns during seizures.

Fundi The posterior, or retinal, surfaces of the eyes.

Gamete Germ cell; egg or sperm. Contains 23 chromosomes, the haploid number.

Gene Localized sequence of DNA specifying one function, usually one protein molecule.

Genetics The science of heredity and variation.

Harelip, cleft lip A lip that is congenitally split or cleft.

Hematoma Blood clot.

Hemiparesis Neurologically speaking, this refers to weakness of one-half of the body.

Hemiplegia Paralysis of one side of the body.

Heredity Resemblance among individuals related by descent; transmission of traits from parents to offspring.

Heterozygous An organism whose chromosomes carry nonidentical genes on any given pair of alleles; possessing different genes in regard to a certain characteristic, eg, hair and brown hair.

Homologous chromosomes The two members of a pair (sister chromosomes).

Homozygote (homozygous) An organism whose chromosomes carry identical genes on any given pair of alleles. The gametes are therefore all alike with respect to this locus, possessing genes for only one member for a pair of characteristics, eg, light, dark; tall, short.

Hyperglycemia High, or elevated blood sugar.

Hyperuricemia   A condition marked by an excess of circulating uric acid in the blood.

Hypocalcemia   Low blood calcium.

Hypoglycemia   Low blood sugar.

Hypoplasia   An incomplete development or defective undergrowth of cells, tissues, or organs.

Hyporeflexia   A weakening of the reflexes.

Hypsarrhythmia   An abnormal, diffusely spiked EEG pattern.

Idiopathic   Unknown as to cause.

Inborn error of metabolism   An inherited disorder due to absence of an enzyme which results in a metabolic block. Usually occurs as recessive traits.

Intelligence quotient—IQ   A computed figure describing a person's intelligence in comparison with performance judged to be normal for a given age.

Karyotype   The appearance of the metaphase chromosomes of an individual or species showing the comparative size, shape, and morphology of the different chromosomes. Usually a photographic representation of the chromosomes arranged in a standard form complying with international standards of nomenclature.

Kernicterus   A condition characterized by deep yellow staining of certain centers of the brain caused by an elevated circulating level of bilirubin in the blood. This causes a widespread neural destruction resulting in severe retardation or death.

Locus (loci)   A fixed position on a chromosome occupied by a given gene or one of its alleles.

Macrocephaly   A condition marked by an exceptionally large head—not necessarily a large brain.

Mainstreaming   An educational concept of placing handicapped children in regular classrooms. It is felt that the delayed child benefits from the social interaction with regular children and from the enriched educational environment, while the normal children benefit by learning to interact with handicapped children early in life.

Malocclusion   A misalignment of the upper and lower teeth.

Meiosis   The process by which the chromosome number of a reproductive (germ) cell becomes reduced to half the diploid (2—) or somatic number. Meiosis results in the formation of gametes in animals, or of spores in plants; it is an important source of variability through recombination.

Meningitis An infection of the meninges, or fibrous coverings of the brain and spinal cord.

Metaphase Stage of cell division in which chromosomes are contracted and have two chromatids. Mitotic metaphase chromosomes are used in karyotyping.

Microcephaly A condition characterized by a small, poorly developed brain, usually associated with a small skull.

Micrognathia A congenital abnormality in size of the jaw, because of markedly reduced bone structure.

Mitosis Cell division in which there is first a duplication of chromosomes followed by migration of chromosomes to the ends of the spindle and dividing of the cytoplasm.

Monosomy State in which one of a pair of chromosomes is missing.

Monozygotic Pertaining to or derived from a single zygote—egg or ovum.

Mosaic An organism, part of which is made up of tissue genetically different from the remaining part.

Motor Neurologically speaking, this refers to muscle activity.

Multifocal Multiple focal areas, as in EEG tracings. Discharges may be identified in multiple but separate areas of brain distribution.

Mutagen An environmental agent, either physical or chemical, that is capable of inducing mutations.

Mutation A permanent heritable change in a gene.

Myoclonus In reference to seizures, single or repetitive jerking movements of small groups of muscles.

Neonatal An age period from birth to one month of age.

Neural tube The embryological forerunner of the central nervous system. It is one of the first identifiable structures to be formed in the embryo, during the fourth week of gestation.

Nondisjunction Failure of homologous paired chromosomes to separate in meiosis. This is the most frequent cause of trisomies.

Occiput The back part of the cranial vault.

Pathogenesis Refers to the cause or developmental process of the pathologic or disease entity.

Pedigree A table, chart, or diagram representing the ancestral history of an individual.

Penetrance Genetically speaking, this refers to the degree in which an abnormal gene is expressed in a hereditary disease process.

Phenotype Physically demonstrable manifestations of a genetic trait.

Phenylketonuria A hereditary amino acid disease commonly called PKU.

Placenta An organ developed in the uterus by the fertilized egg, which serves to supply food and nutrition to the fetus and remove waste products. The afterbirth.

Polydactyly A condition marked by the presence of more fingers and/or toes than normal.

Polygenic Many genes, each with a small additive effect on the phenotype; usually used to indicate the involvement of many genes.

Postictal The period of time immediately after a seizure.

Prognosis The medical judgment as to the probable course of a patient's disease and prospects for recovery.

Proximal-distal development The growth process observed in children in which the child gains control of the areas of his body which are close to his trunk (ie, his shoulders and hips) before he gains control of his hands and feet.

Psychomotor Muscle or motor behavioral activity relating to complex sequences or patterns of behavior.

Psychosis Severe mental disorder characterized by a loss of contact with reality.

Seizure An episode of involuntary muscle and/or sensory activity characterized by sudden onset and offset and associated with abnormal electrical discharges in brain wave tracings.

Sex chromosomes Chromosomes that are particularly connected with the determination of sex.

Sex-linked Carried on the X chromosomes; X-linked is a more specific term. Most sex-linked diseases find overt expression only in males.

Subdural This refers to the space between the dura and the arachnoid membranes, both of which are part of the meninges or fibrous coverings of the brain and spinal cord.

Syndrome A group of symptoms that occur together and represent a particular disease.

Temporal lobe One of the major lobular divisions of the cerebrum and one which appears particularly susceptible to epileptogenic activity. The others are the frontal, parietal, and occipital lobes.

Teratogenic Capable of producing malformations during embryonic development.

Tomogram An x-ray of a selected layer of the body.

Tonic Refers to increased muscle tone or rigidity during seizure activity.

Toxoplasmosis A benign infection by a rickettsial agent which, if present during embryologic and fetal development, can cause malformations of brain and body development.

Translocation Displacement of part or all of one chromosome onto another. If the total amount of genetic material is unchanged, it is referred to as a balanced translocation.

Trisomy Three rather than two members of a given chromosome are present.

Trypsin-Giemsa banding Special staining technique which reveals chromosomal bands. Allows for the identification of all human chromosomes. Similar in principle to fluorescent banding which it has largely superceded.

Tuberous sclerosis An inherited disease state manifest by slow growing tumor development in the skin, brain, and abdominal viscera (liver, kidneys, spleen). It is dominantly inherited and has low penetrance.

Ultrasound, ultrasonography The laboratory procedure which visualizes the deep structures of the body by recording the reflection of ultrasonic waves directed into the tissues.

Uterus The saclike structure in which the embryo of mammals develops within the mother's body.

X-linked See sex-linked.

Zygote The earliest product of conception, formed when the sperm and the egg unite.

APPENDIX 2

SERVICES FOR HANDICAPPED CHILDREN
AND THEIR FAMILIES

Many organizations can offer useful information and services to handicapped children and their families. A complete listing can be found in The Directory of National Information Sources of Handicapping Conditions and Related Services, Clearinghouse on the Handicapped, Office for Handicapped Individuals, DHEW, Washington, DC 20201. This directory should be available in most large centers for the handicapped. The following list gives a brief description of the services available through some of these organizations.

American Foundation for the Blind, 15 West 16th Street, New York, NY 10011. The foundation provides reading materials, refers clients to local service agencies, and sells aids and appliances for blind persons. Membership and subscription to *The AFB Newsletter* are free.

Association for Children with Learning Disabilities, 4156 Library Road, Pittsburgh, PA 15234. A national association with local affiliates in 50 states. A free information packet provides information on learning disabilities, parents' rights, and other resources available.

Closer Look Information Center, Box 1492, Washington, DC 20013. A project of the federal government's Bureau of Education for the Handicapped. Closer Look provides, free of charge, packets of information giving practical advice to parents of handicapped children. When you write to Closer Look, indicate the nature of your child's handicap—mental retardation plus any other associated condition, such as deafness or cerebral palsy. The center will send names of government and private agencies in your area, reading lists, information on educational rights and opportunities, and other material relating to your child's specific handicap. A newsletter, *Report from Closer Look,* also is available.

Epilepsy Foundation of America, 1828 L Street NW, Suite 406, Washington, DC 20036. The Foundation and its 90 affiliates provide reading material, self-help groups, and a low-cost, mail-order prescription service. Annual dues include subscription to the newsletter, *National Spokesman.*

Exceptional Parent, 20 Providence Street, Room 708, Boston, MA 02116. This national bimonthly magazine offers practical guidance to parents of disabled children, including the mentally retarded.

National Association for Retarded Citizens (NARC) 2709 Avenue E East, Arlington, TX 76011. NARC, the major private organization for mentally retarded persons and their families, is engaged in a number of services—education, research, advocacy, counseling, and others.

Membership in the 50 state and 1800 local groups consists mainly of parents but also includes professional workers and other interested people. Your state or local affiliate can provide information on services available in your area, such as respite care (home care during family emergencies and vacations), special camps, infant stimulation programs, sheltered workshops, and community homes. Request a copy of the NARC "Publications List," which offers numerous helpful booklets for nominal fees. Membership fees depend on the local chapter; subscription to *Mental Retardation News* is included.

National Association of the Deaf, 814 Thayer Avenue, Silver Spring, MD 20910. This association, through its 47 state affiliates, offers informational assistance, legal services, an insurance program, and advocacy. Membership dues include a subscription to the association's magazine, *The Deaf American.*

National Easter Seal Society for Crippled Children and Adults, 2023 West Ogden Avenue, Chicago, IL 60612. The National Easter Seal Society provides a multitude of direct services to the handicapped people through its 52 state and 2000 local groups. Your local society may offer some of the following: information, referral, and follow-up; infant stimulation, and preschool programs; speech, hearing, physical, occupational, and rehabilitation therapy; homebound craft programs; vocational evaluations, sheltered workshops, and job placement; camping and other recreational and social activities; vocational, personal adjustment, and parent counseling; housing; transportation; and dental services. Many local affiliates open their programs to mentally retarded persons who are not physically handicapped. Services are provided free or are charged according to the client's ability to pay. The national society has many practical publications (including a directory of special camps) available at a nominal cost. Its newsletter, *Easter Seal Communicator,* is free.

National Foundation—March of Dimes, P.O. Box 2000, White Plains, NY 10602. This national organization provides bulletins, pamphlets on rubella, birth defects, and drugs. They also provide lists of genetic counseling centers and medical services. Local chapters can usually be found in the white pages of the telephone book.

National Information and Referral Service for Autistic and Autisticlike Persons, 306 31st Street, Huntington, WV 25702. A free information package and referrals to facilities, programs, and services are available. For membership in the National Society for Autistic Children, Inc., write to the Society, 621 Central Avenue, Albany, NY 12206. Annual membership includes subscription to NSAC Newsletter.

Parents of Children with Down's Syndrome, c/o Northern Virginia Association for Retarded Citizens, 105 East Annandale Road, Suite 203, Falls Church, VA 22046. This organization provides a kit of informational material on Down syndrome, article reprints, and a reading list for a small fee.

President's Committee on Mental Retardation, Washington, DC 20201. This committee offers an information and referral service and has numerous publications available, either free or for a nominal charge. Services to parents also consist of a telephone information service (202) 245-7520, which can help answer your general and specific questions, including those concerning legal and civil rights of mentally retarded persons. The committee's monthly newsletter, *News Break,* is free.

Spina Bifida Association of America, 343 South Dearborn Street, Suite 319, Chicago, IL 60604. Free informational brochures, several inexpensive booklets, and a referral to one of 73 state and local chapters are among the services offered by this association. Membership: varies among local chapters; subscription to the newsletter, *Pipeline,* is extra.

United Cerebral Palsy Associations, 66 East 34th Street, New York, NY 10016. The 260 state and local affiliates of United Cerebral Palsy offer care, treatment, and training to children and adults with cerebral palsy; related services are provided to their families. In some areas, a mentally retarded person who does not have cerebral palsy may qualify for services. Informational booklets and subscriptions to two newsletters, *Word from Washington* and *UCP Crusader,* are free. Membership: nominal, depending upon the local chapter.

US Department of Health, Education, and Welfare, Alcohol and Drug Abuse Bureau, USDHEW, Washington, DC 20201. This Bureau provides free informational brochures and referral information in the area of alcoholism and drug abuse. There have been some recent publications on the fetal alcohol syndrome and smoking and the fetus which are available from this Bureau.

OTHER SERVICES

Information and referral
    State developmental disability agency or state department of mental health
    County health department
    Regional clinic for mentally retarded persons

Infant stimulation programs/advice on management
    State developmental disability agency or state department of mental health
    County health department
    Regional clinic
    Public health nursing association

Education (including preschool)
    State department of special education
    Regional clinic

College or university special education department
Principal or special education director of local school
Nursery schools
Public and private day-care centers
Churches

Respite care
State division of family services
County health department
Homemaker/health aide agencies

Recreation
Public schools
City recreation department
Scouting programs
YMCA and YWCAs
Churches
Special camps
American Red Cross swimming program
Special Olympics

Rehabilitation, jobs, and community residential facilities
State developmental disability agency or state department of mental
    health
State department of vocational rehabilitation
Special education department of colleges and universities
Special education director of local school

Financial
US Social Security Administration
Title XIX (Medicaid)
State developmental disability agency or state department of mental
    health
Veterans' services
State crippled children's programs
Vocational rehabilitation services
Armed Forces medical services
Private health insurance
Religious group social and welfare services

SUGGESTED READINGS

Alcohol Abuse

Alcohol and Your Unborn Baby. DHEW Pub. No. (ADM) 78-521, National Institute on Alcohol Abuse and Addiction. Rockville, Md.: Public Health Service.

Birth Defects

Bergsma, D. (Ed.). *Birth Defects Compendium,* 2nd Ed. New York: Alan R. Liss, 1979.

Child Development

Apgar, V., and Beck, J. *Is My Baby All Right? A Guide to Birth Defects.* New York: Trident, 1972.

Christopherson, E.R. *Little People: Guidelines for Common Sense Child Rearing.* Lawrence, Kans.: H. & H. Enterprises, 1977.

Klaus, M.H., and Kennell, J.H. *Maternal-Infant Bonding.* St. Louis: C.V. Mosby, 1976.

La Leche League. *The Womanly Art of Breast Feeding.*

Warner, M.P. *A Doctor Discusses Breast Feeding.* Chicago: Budlong Press, 1970.

Down Syndrome

Hanson, M.J. *Teaching Your Down's Syndrome Infant: A Guide for Parents.* Eugene, Ore.: University of Oregon, 1977.

Hunt, N. *The World of Nigel Hunt: The Diary of a Mongoloid Youth.* New York: Taplinger Publishing Company, 1967.

Koch, R., and de la Cruz, F.F. *Down's Syndrome (Mongolism).* New York: Bruner/Mazel, 1975.

Pueschel, S.M., et al. *Down's Syndrome: Growing and Learning.* Kansas City: Sheed, Andrews, and McMeel, 1978.

Roberts, N., and Roberts, B. *David.* Richmond, Va.: John Knox Press, 1968.

Smith, D.W., and Wilson, A.A. *The Child with Down's Syndrome (Mongolism).* Philadelphia: W.B. Saunders, 1973.

Smith, G.F., and Berg, J.M. *Down's Anomaly.* Edinburgh: Churchill Livingstone, 1976.

Emotional Disorders

Becker, W.C. *Parents Are Teachers.* Champaign, Ill.: Research Press, 1971.

Bell, T.H. *Your Child's Intellect—A Guide to Home-Based Preschool Education.* Salt Lake City: Olympus Publishing Company, 1973.

Bradley, C. *Schizophrenia in Childhood.* New York: Macmillan, 1941.

Della-Piana, G. *How to Talk with Children (and Other People).* New York: John Wiley, 1973.

Dreikurs, R. *Coping With Children's Misbehavior: A Parent's Guide.* New York: Hawthorn Books, 1972.

Dreikurs, R., and Cassel, P. *Discipline Without Tears.* New York: Hawthorn Books, 1972.

Dreikurs, R., and Grey, L. *A Parent's Guide to Child Discipline.* New York: Hawthorn Books, 1970.

Dreikurs, R., and Soltz, V. *Children: The Challenge.* New York: Hawthorn Books, 1964.

Ginott, H.G. *Between Parent and Child.* New York: Avon Books, 1955.

Ginott, H.G. *Between Parent and Teenager.* New York: Avon Books, 1969.

Gordon, T. *Parent Effectiveness Training.* New York: P.H. Wyden, 1970.

Kanner, L. Autistic disturbances of affective contact. *Nervous Child* 2:217–300, 1943.

Kanner, L. Follow-up study of eleven autistic children originally reported in 1943. *J Autism Child Schiz.* 1:119–145, 1971.

Kessler, J.W. *Psychopathology of Childhood.* Englewood Cliffs, N.J.: Prentice-Hall, 1966.

Krumbholtz, J.D., and Krumbholtz, H.B. *Changing Children's Behavior.* Englewood Cliffs, N.J.: Prentice-Hall, 1972.

O'Leary, K.D., and Wilson, S.T. *Behavior Therapy: Application and Outcome.* Englewood Cliffs, N.J.: Prentice-Hall, 1975.

Patterson, G.R. *Living With Children.* Champaign, Ill.: Research Press, 1976.

Phillips, E.L. Contributions to a learning theory account of childhood autism. Edited by E.P. Trapp, and P. Himelstein. In *Readings on the Exceptional Child.* New York: Appleton-Century-Crofts, 1962.

Epilepsy

Aird, R.B., and Woodbury, D. *The Management of Epilepsy.* Springfield, Ill.: Charles C Thomas, 1974.

Baird, H.W. *The Child with Convulsions: A Guide for Parents, Teachers, Counselors, and Medical Personnel.* New York: Grune and Stratton, 1972.

Kemp, R.P. *Understanding Epilepsy.* London: Tavistock, 1963.

Kreindler, A. *Legal Rights of Persons with Epilepsy.* Washington, D.C.: Epilepsy Foundation of America, 1972.

Livingston, S. *Comprehensive Management of Epilepsy in Infancy, Childhood and Adolescence.* Springfield, Ill.: Charles C Thomas, 1971.

Lunt, C.P. *How to Live with Epilepsy.* New York: Twayne, 1961.

Scott, D.F. *About Epilepsy,* Revised Ed. New York: International Universities, 1973.

Genetics

De Grouchy, J., and Turleau, C. *Clinical Atlas of Human Chromosomes.* New York: John Wiley, 1977.

Fraser-Roberts, J.A. *An Introduction to Medical Genetics,* 6th Ed. New York: Oxford University Press, 1973.

McKusick, V.A. *Mendelian Inheritance in Man. Catalogs of Autosomal Dominant, Autosomal Recessive, and X-Linked Phenotypes,* 5th Ed. Baltimore: Johns Hopkins University Press, 1978.

Milunsky, A. *The Prevention of Genetic Disease and Mental Retardation.* Philadelphia: W.B. Saunders, 1975.

Milunsky, A. *Know Your Genes.* Boston: Houghton-Mifflin, 1977.

Milunsky, A., and Annas, G.J. (Eds.). *Genetics and the Law.* New York: Plenum Press, 1976.

Riccardi, V.M. *The Genetic Approach to Human Disease.* New York: Oxford University Press, 1977.

Thompson, J.S., and Thompson, M.W. *Genetics in Medicine,* 2nd Ed. Philadelphia: W.B. Saunders, 1973.

Zellweger, H., and Simpson, J. *Chromosomes of Man.* Philadelphia: J.B. Lippincott, 1977.

Intellectual Development

Becker, W.C., Englemann, S., and Thomas, D.R. *Cognitive Learning and Instruction.* Chicago: Science Research Associates, 1975.

234

Bradley, R.H., and Caldwell, B.M. Early home environment and changes in mental test performance in children from 6 to 36 months. *Developmental Psychology* 12:93–97, 1976.

McCall, R.B., Appelbaum, M.I., and Hogarty, P.S. Developmental changes in mental performance. *Monogr Soc Res Child Devel.* 38:3, 1973.

Phillips, J.L. *Origins of Intellect: Piaget's Theory.* San Francisco: W.H. Freeman, 1969.

Language Development

Chomsky, N. Language training. Edited by J.P.B. Allen and P. Van Buren. In *Chomsky Selected Readings.* New York: Oxford University Press, 1971.

Gray, B.B., and Ryan, B.P. *A Language Program for the Nonlanguage Child.* Champaign, Ill.: Research Press, 1973.

Lenneberg, E. *Biological Foundations of Language.* New York: John Wiley, 1967.

Ruder, K., and Smith, M.D. Issues in language training. Edited by R.L. Schiefelbusch, and L.L. Lloyd. In *Language Perspectives: Acquisition, Retardation, and Intervention.* Baltimore: University Park Press, 1974.

Malformations—Abnormal Development

Bergsma, D. (Ed.). *Birth Defects Atlas and Compendium.* Baltimore: Williams and Wilkins, 1973.

Rimoin, D.L. The chondrodystrophies. Edited by H. Harris, and K. Hirschorn. In *Advances in Human Genetics,* Vol. V. New York: Plenum Press, 1975.

Smith, D.W. *Patterns of Human Malformation.* Philadelphia: W.B. Saunders, 1970.

MBD—Hyperactivity—Learning Disabilities

Adler, S.J. *Your Overactive Child.* New York: Medcom Press, 1972.

Brady, J.P., and Brodie, H.K. (Eds.). *CNS Activating Drugs in the Treatment of the Hyperactive Child. Controversy in Psychiatry.* Philadelphia: W.B. Saunders, 1978.

Cantwell, D.P. *The Hyperactive Child: Diagnosis, Management, and Current Research.* New York: Spectrum, 1975.

Millichap, J.G. *The Hyperactive Child with Minimal Brain Dysfunction.* New York: Year Book, 1975.

Safer, D.J., and Allen, R.P. *Hyperactive Children: Diagnosis and Management.* Baltimore: University Park Press, 1976.

Wender, P.H. *The Hyperactive Child—A Handbook for Parents.* New York: Crown, 1973.

Wender, P.H. *Minimal Brain Dysfunction in Children.* New York: Wiley-Interscience, 1971.

Mental Retardation

Crome, L., and Stern, J. *Pathology of Mental Retardation,* 2nd Ed. Baltimore: Williams and Wilkins, 1972.

Ehlers, W.H., Krishef, C.H., and Prothero, J.C. *An Introduction to Mental Retardation—A Programmed Text,* 2nd Ed. Columbus: Mo. Merrill, 1977.

Holmes, L.B., et al. *Mental Retardation: An Atlas of Diseases with Associated Physical Abnormalities.* New York: Macmillan, 1972.

Manual on Terminology and Classification in Mental Retardation. American Association of Mental Diseases, 1977.

Metabolic Errors

Bondy, P.K., and Rosenberg, L.E. (Eds.). *Duncan's Disease of Metabolism,* Vol. 1, 7th Ed. Philadelphia: W.B. Saunders, 1974.

Stanbury, J.B., Wyngaarden, J.B., Frederickson, D.S. (Eds.). *The Metabolic Basis of Inherited Disease,* 3rd Ed. New York: McGraw-Hill, 1972.

Motor/Physical Growth and Development

Caplan, F. (Ed.). *The Parenting Advisor.* Garden City, N.Y.: Anchor Books, 1978.

Connor, F.P., Williamson, G.G., and Siepp, J.M. *Program Guide for Infants and Toddlers with Neuromuscular and Other Developmental Disabilities.* New York: Teachers College Press, 1978.

Finnie, N. *Handling the Young Cerebral Palsied Child at Home.* New York: E.P. Dutton, 1975.

Holle, B. *Motor Development in Children: Normal and Retarded.* Oxford: Blackwell Scientific Pub., 1976.

236

Self-Help

Ainsworth, M.D., and Bell, W.M. Some contemporary patterns of mother-infant interaction in the feeding situation. Edited by J.H. Ambrose. In *Stimulation in Early Infancy.* London: Academic Press, 1969.

Carlson, N. (Ed.). *The Context of Life: A Socio-ecological Model of Adaptive Behavior and Functioning.* East Lansing, Mich.: Michigan State University, 1976.

Clark-Stewart, K.A. Interactions between mothers and their young children: characteristics and consequences. *Monogr Soc Res Child Devel.* 38:6-7, 1973.

Sensory and Perceptual Development

Gibson, E.J., and Walls, R.D. The effect of prolonged exposure to visually present patterns or learning to discriminate them. *J Comp Physiol Psychol.* 49:239-242, 1956.

Uzgiris, I.C. Ordanility in the development of schemas for relating to objects. Edited by J. Hellmuth. In *The Exceptional Infant.* Seattle: Special Child Publications, Vol. I. 1967.

White, G.L., and Castle, P.W. Visual exploratory behavior following post-natal handling of human infants. *Percept Mot Skills.* 18:497-502, 1964.

Social-Emotional

Bowlby, J. *Attachment and Loss.* New York: Basic Books, 1969.

Bromwich, R.M. Stimulation in the first year of life: a perspective on infant development. *Young Children* 32:71-82, 1977.

Casto, G., et al. *Affective Behavior in Preschool Children.* Logan, Utah: Utah State University, 1976.

Schaffer, H.R. *The Growth of Sociability.* Middlesex, England: Penguin Books, 1971.

Stechler, G., and Carpenter, G. A viewpoint on early affective development. Edited by J. Hellmuth. In *The Exceptional Infant.* New York: Bruner/Mazel, 1967.

Turner Syndrome

Plumridge, D., *Good Things Come in Small Packages—The Whys and Hows of Turner's Syndrome.* Eugene. Ore.: University of Oregon, 1976.

APPENDIX 4

ANNOTATED BIBLIOGRAPHY

The descriptions of the following books are excerpted from the Parent Resource Library through the courtesy of the Outreach and Development Division of the Exceptional Child Center at Utah State University, Logan, Utah.

The Parent Resource Library is a free service for parents of handicapped children in the four-state area of Utah, Idaho, Wyoming, and Nevada. This catalog is a listing of some books and pamphlets available from the Library. Books are listed according to subject. Books are listed in sequence, according to reading difficulty or content level.

For additional information, please contact: Parent Resource Library, Exceptional Child Center, UMC 68, Utah State University, Logan, Utah 84322.

BEHAVIOR MANAGEMENT

Living With Children by Gerald R. Patterson. Champaign, Ill.: Resarch Press, 1968. Programmed book. Situations are given and reader fills in appropriate word. Answers at bottom of page. Emphasizes methods other than punishment to change undesirable behavior. For example, social and nonsocial reinforcers can be used. Describes how parents and children learn from each other. Spanish edition available upon request. Content level: Moderately easy.

Parent Effectiveness Training by Thomas Gordon. New York: Peter H. Wyden, 1970. Complete process of learning how to communicate with children and develop mutual respect. Teaches active listening, "I-messages," and problem-solving. Many communities offer courses on this book. Content level: Intermediate.

Changing Children's Behavior by John D. and Helen B. Krumbholtz. Englewood Cliffs, N.J.: Prentice-Hall, 1972. Many examples of inappropriate and appropriate behavior given. Emphasis on positive reinforcement, rather than punishment. Examples of how people reinforce behaviors they do not want and do not know they are using. Tells how to weaken inappropriate behavior. Some information on dealing with fear in children. Content level: Intermediate.

Children: The Challenge by Rudolf Dreikurs and Vicki Soltz. New York: Hawthorn Books, 1964. Many specific examples of parent and child behavior given. Emphasis on consistency and establishing mutual respect. Firmness without being domineering. Avoid lecturing the child. Use of natural and logical consequences. Content level: Intermediate.

237

SPECIFIC PROBLEMS

Some Special Problems of Children: Aged Two to Five Years by Nina Ridenour and Isabel Johnson. New York: Child Study Association of America, 1966. Book takes special problems, such as destructiveness, bad language, and thumbsucking, and looks at each separately. Suggestions given on how to correct problem. Goes into the "whys" of certain behaviors. Content level: Moderately Easy.

A Handicapped Child in the Family: A Guide for Parents by Verda Heisler. New York: Grune and Stratton, 1972. Although written about a therapy group made up of parents of cerebral palsied children, it is appropriate for any parent of a handicapped child. Written about the sessions over a period of two years. Shows the changes in attitudes and development of thinking of the parents, who slowly learn to express the resentment, hostility, and real feelings and fears, and learn how to deal with them. Content level: Intermediate.

The Hyperactive Child: A Handbook for Parents by Paul Wender. Pittsburgh, Penn.: Association for Children With Learning Disabilities, 1973. Complete discussion on hyperactive children—characteristics, treatment and medication (which drugs are for what). Much of the book is devoted to understanding the hyperactive child. Content level: Moderately Difficult.

BOOKS FOR BROTHERS AND SISTERS
OF HANDICAPPED PERSONS

The Summer of the Swans by Betsy Byars. New York: Viking Press, 1972. A story about a girl of many moods trying to enjoy the summer and be happy with herself the way she is. She has a mentally retarded brother named Charlie, who disappears one night. In trying to find him, Sara gains insight into herself. Content level: Moderately Easy.

CEREBRAL PALSY

So Your Child Has Cerebral Palsy by Gil S. Joel. Albuquerque, N.M.: University of New Mexico Press, 1975. Problems parents of cerebral palsied children face discussed by a cerebral palsied person who counsels handicapped people. Good insight into the needs of the cerebral palsied, and suggestions on how parents can meet those needs. Content level: Moderately Easy.

Handling the Young Cerebral Palsied Child at Home by Nancie R. Finnie. New York: E.P. Dutton and Co., 1968. Excellent book. Very complete and factual. Detailed descriptions of problems with each major type of cerebral palsy, and what to do about it. Emphasis on physical movement—how to hold, pick up, carry, etc. Very specific. Helpful to parents or professionals. Content level: Intermediate.

DEVELOPING LEARNING AT HOME

Teach Your Baby by Genevieve Painter. New York: Simon and Schuster, 1971. Designed for infants and young children, from birth to three years. Many detailed stimulation activities for infants. Activities arranged by monthly age of child. Many drawings and specific directions. Excellent for new parents. Content level: Moderately Difficult.

Your Child's Intellect—A Guide to Home-Based Preschool by T.H. Bell. Salt Lake City: Olympus Pub. Co., 1973. Very motivating format. Lots of pictures. Instructions and directions arranged for easy reading. Program designed for preschoolers from birth to five years. Sequenced activities to stimulate and motivate child. Content level: Intermediate.

Child Learning Through Child Play: Learning Activities for 2- and 3-Year-Olds by Ira Gordon, et al. New York: St. Martin Press, 1972. Learning activities for two- and three-year-olds, could go up to five-year-olds. Specific instructions for ideas and things to do. Limited number of activities. Some drawings. Content level: Intermediate.

IMPAIRED HEARING

Home Screening for Hearing Disorders in Infants by Speech Pathology, Audiology Section, Department of Social Services, Salt Lake City, Utah, 1976. A four-part test, using objects found at home, like baby food jars and popcorn. Basic idea: shake object behind child's head and see if he hears it. Can be performed easily by parent. Content level: Moderately Easy.

Hearing-Impaired Preschool Child: A Book for Parents by Jean E. Semple. Springfield, Ill.: Charles C Thomas, 1970. Discusses many problems of having a hearing-impaired child, such as discipline communication, toilet training, attitudes and guilt of parents and community. What hearing aids can and cannot do, how to care for them, language and speech development. Gives development of the normal child from six months to five years. Twelve lessons for parents to do at home on a daily basis. Content level: Moderately Difficult.

DOWN SYNDROME

The Child with Down's Syndrome by David W. Smith and Ann Asper Wilson. Philadelphia: W.B. Saunders, 1973. Lots of pictures of

Down children from birth through adulthood. Very pleasing format. Cause of Down syndrome discussed in detail with drawings of genes and chromosomes. Characteristics of Down syndrome shown through pictures. Emphasis on the problems of the family of a Down syndrome child and their adjustment. Personal experiences and comments from parents. Content level: Intermediate.

Teaching Your Down's Syndrome Infant: A Guide for Parents by Marci J. Hanson. Eugene, Ore.: Center on Human Development, University of Oregon, 1977. A manual designed for parents of Down syndrome infants or for professionals working with the parents. Covers birth to two years. Teaching programs are concerned with motor skills.

David by Nancy Roberts and Bruce Roberts. Richmond, Virginia: John Knox Press, 1974. The first four years in the life of a Down syndrome boy as documented by his parents. The text by his mother and the photographs by his father tell the story of the development of a happy, sensitive, "different" child, and the problems and feelings of his parents during those early years. Content level: Moderately Easy.

MENTALLY RETARDED

You and Your Retarded Child by Samuel A. Kirk, Merle B. Karnes, and Winifred Kirk. Palo Alto, Calif.: Pacific Books, 1968. Excellent listing of expected behaviors at specified age levels for normal children with instructions given parents on how to figure out the degree of their child's retardation. Written for parents in lay terms—not technical. Good suggestions for parents to help teach their child self-help skills, talking, behavior control. Content level: Intermediate.

Manual on Terminology and Classification in Mental Retardation by the American Association on Mental Deficiency, 1977. This manual contains the official terminology and classification on mental retardation as proposed by the American Association on Mental Deficiency. It also contains a discussion of classification based on IQ scores and adaptive behavior scales. A complete listing of adaptive behavior scales is included.

PHYSICALLY HANDICAPPED

Is My Baby All Right? A Guide to Birth Defects by Virginia Apgar and Joan Beck. New York: Trident Press, Division of Simon and Schuster, 1972. Begins with specific information on fetal development, genetics and heredity, how and when birth defects may begin, preventing birth defects, pregnancy and delivery. Rest of the book discusses many different types of handicaps. Useful for couples who want children, expectant mothers, or parents who want to find out more about a handicap. Very complete. Content level: Moderately Difficult.

RECREATION

Recreation for the Mentally Retarded by Southern Regional Education Board. Atlanta, Ga., 1964. Written for ward personnel in institutions, but also applicable for parents. Many games and activities listed for groups and individuals. Includes equipment needed, how many can play and instructions. Areas covered: active games, music and rhythms, quiet games and table games, arts and crafts, homemade games and equipment. Content level: Moderately Easy.

Play Activities for the Retarded Child by Bernice Wells Carlson and David R. Ginglend. Nashville, Tenn.: Abington Press, 1961. Book covers many activities divided into five major areas: mental health, social, physical, language, and intellectual. Activities in order of difficulty in each area. Begins with defining the need to play. Activities in these areas: informal and imaginative play, follow the leader and choral speaking, table work and games, learning handicraft skills, handicraft for special reasons, music and other games. Content level: Intermediate.

SEX EDUCATION

How to Tell Your Child About Sex by James L. Humes, Jr. New York: Public Affairs Pamphlets, 1979. How to answer children's questions about sex and talk to them about it openly. Would be good for parent just beginning to think about it or for new parent. Content level: Intermediate.

Facts About Sex for Today's Youth by Sol Gordon. New York: John Day Co., 1973. Basic information on reproductive systems, intercourse, pregnancy, birth, contraception, sex problems. Good as background for parents. Excellent for late elementary or early junior high kids. Many good illustrations. Easy format reading level. Content level: Moderately Easy.

SPEECH AND LANGUAGE

Getting Your Baby Ready to Talk by John Tracy Clinic. Los Angeles, 1968. Curriculum for use at home and by parents. Lessons are sequenced. Many activities and ideas for parents. Lessons are color-coded throughout. Content level: Moderately Easy.

Teach Your Child to Talk by the staff of the Developmental Language and Speech Center. New York: Cebco Publ. Co., 1957. Many specific ideas and activities for parents. Format: Activities arranged by months of development, birth to six months, six to 12 months, etc. Goes to five years. Appendix contains speech sounds, finger plays, books for children, books for parents. No discussion on handicapped children. Content level: Intermediate.

Your Developmentally Retarded Child Can Communicate by Julia S. Molloy and Arlene Matkin. New York: John Day Co., 1975. A guide for parents and teachers in speech, language, and nonverbal communication. Progresses from basic principles of speech and other means of communication to specific steps to follow in working with children. Quite a bit of reading required to get the information, but the ideas are good. Content level: Intermediate.

For the Parents of a Child Whose Speech is Delayed by R. Corbin Pennington and Elizabeth James. Danville, Ill.: Interstate Printers and Publ., 1965. Emphasis on talking with children. General information on all children's speech development. Causes of delayed speech: low intelligence, brain damage, hearing loss, illness, poor speech at home, accidents or shock, no need for speech, conflict in the home, poor teaching. Content level: Intermediate.

TRAINING IN SELF-HELP SKILLS

Toilet Training in Less Than a Day by Nathan H. Azrin and Richard M. Foxx. New York: Simon and Schuster, 1974. Written for normal children. Very effective procedures—use a doll that wets as an example, place potty chair in kitchen, lots of liquids and treats. Much praise used. Punishment—child must clean up puddle, touch his wet pants several times, practice lowering and raising pants. Excellent method if child can handle it. Content level: Moderately Difficult.

Toilet Training the Retarded by Richard M. Foxx and Nathan H. Azrin. Champaign, Ill.: Research Press, 1973. Very complete book listing explicit steps and procedures to follow in training the retarded. Excellent for parents or institution personnel. Describes training methods: give the retarded child lots of liquids—wait and talk about wanting dry pants—take to toilet, help remove pants, sit on toilet 20 minutes. If child voids, reward with praise, hug and treat. Maintenance program described. Content level: Difficult.

Help Them Grow! by Jane Blumenfeld, Pearl E. Thompson and Beverly S. Vogel. Nashville, Tenn.: Abington Press, 1971. Pictorial book giving reasons for teaching the mentally retarded child independence and self-help skills. Suggestions for parents. Many areas covered: family-living, self-help, social skills, communication skills, sensory and motor skills. Gives good, basic help. Content level: Easy.

Early Self-Help Skills by Bruce L. Baker, Alan J. Brightman, Louis J. Heifetz, and Diane M. Murphy. Champaign, Ill.: Research Press, 1976. A manual in the series "Steps to Independence, A Skills Training

Series for Children with Special Needs," designed to help parents use time spent with their child effectively. Describes general principles of teaching which parents can adapt to their own style and situation. Also presents step-by-step skill-teaching programs to match the child's ability level. Uses an easy-to-follow format emphasizing self-help readiness skills, basic motor skills, motor activities, eating, dressing, and grooming. Content level: Intermediate.

Intermediate Self-Help Skills by Bruce L. Baker, Alan J. Brightman, Louis J. Heifetz, and Diane M. Murphy. Champaign, Ill.: Research Press, 1976. A manual in the series "Steps to Independence, A Skills Training Series for Children with Special Needs," designed to help parents use time spent with their child effectively. Describes general principles of teaching parents can adapt to their own style and situation and also presents step-by-step skill-teaching programs to match the child's ability level. Uses an easy-to-follow format emphasizing dressing, eating, grooming, and housekeeping skills. Content level: Intermediate.

Advanced Self-Help Skills by Bruce L. Baker, Alan J. Brightman, Louis J. Heifetz, and Diane M. Murphy. Champaign, Ill.: Research Press, 1976. A manual in the series, "Steps to Independence, A Skills Training Series for Children with Special Needs," designed to help parents use time spent with their child effectively. Describes general principles of teaching parents can adapt to their own style and situation and also presents step-by-step skill-teaching programs to match the child's ability level. Uses an easy-to-follow format emphasizing dressing, eating, grooming, and housekeeping skills. Content level: Intermediate.

IMPAIRED VISION

Blind Pre-School by Billie M. Taylor. Colorado Springs, Colo.: Industrial Printers of Colorado, 1974. Compilation of various articles that the author felt would be helpful to parents of preschool blind children. Some articles are general in nature, others give specific activities or information on blindness. Content level: Intermediate.

INDEX

MA